PREVENTION OVER PRESCRIPTION

Take Control of Your Health through Nutrition, Movement, and Community

DR. KWADWO KYEREMANTENG

Lucky Book Publishing

To request permissions, contact the publisher at hello@luckybookpublishing.com.

Paperback ISBN: 978-1-998287-65-9
Hardcover ISBN: 978-1-998287-66-6
E-book ISBN: 978-1-998287-67-3

1st edition, May 2025

"If you're ready to stop reacting to symptoms and start taking control, Prevention Over Prescription delivers simple, science-backed strategies to be proactive about your health and biology."

- Ben Azadi, Author of Metabolic Freedom

DEDICATION

To my kids—my greatest inspiration and the core reason I strive to be the best version of myself. My hope is to set an example for you of how to live a healthy, functional, and meaningful life. Love you boys.

To everyone out there still searching for their purpose, struggling to find alignment and direction—this book is for you. Believe me, you will find your path. I truly hope these pages serve you well.

Lastly, to my incredible wife, Cathy. Thank you for giving me the space to dream big, for supporting my passion to serve others, and for holding our family together with unwavering strength. You've stood by me through my lowest moments and celebrated with me at my highest. Love you, Mommie.

MY GIFT TO YOU

I am so glad you're here!

As my Gift to you, get FREE Access to the Audiobook of Prevention Over Prescription and other bonus content by scanning the QR Code below or visiting drkwadwo.ca

Get 15% off your order at Gyata Nutrition by using the code KWADCAST15 at gyatanutrition.com.

Claim your free LMNT sample pack at drinkLMNT.com/kwadcast.

Interested in personalized coaching or advisory services?
Visit my coaching page at drkwadwo.ca/advisory to learn more.

TABLE OF CONTENTS

INTRODUCTION
THE POWER OF PREVENTION

"My focus now is upstream—empowering people to take control of their health before they end up in crisis."
– Dr. Kwadwo Kyeremanteng

The ICU is a place where critical decisions are made to save lives. One of the most rewarding experiences anyone could have is being there for people when they need it most. As an ICU doctor, I've spent my career at the forefront of life-and-death situations. However, over the years, one truth has become painfully clear to me: If someone ends up in the ICU, their chances of a full recovery or returning to their previous level of function are often slim. The road back is long, even when we manage to save lives, as many never fully regain what they lost. Also, the physical and emotional toll on patients and their families is immense, and it often becomes a turning point in their lives, but not in the way they would hope.

Reflecting on my career, I've realized that while the ICU can save lives, it's not where the battle for health should begin. For years, healthcare has focused on treating disease symptoms rather than addressing the root causes. This approach is reactive, dealing with issues only after they have become critical. It's akin to putting out fires without ever asking why the fires started in the first place. This mindset, deeply ingrained in the healthcare system, often leaves us chasing after solutions when it's too late.

On the flip side, my career has also been filled with the constant search for the best treatments—whether it's deciding which fluids to use, which products to prioritize, or how to save a few extra dollars in healthcare costs. These decisions are critical but often feel like putting band-aids on more significant problems. The more I delved into this, especially during the COVID-19 pandemic, the more I realized we were missing something crucial, as we primarily focused on treating illness and neglected the power of prevention. We were fighting battles that could have been avoided altogether.

COVID-19 was a wake-up call for the world and a stark reminder for me as a physician. It exposed the quietly growing vulnerabilities in our health that have been mainly left unchecked for years. The disease targeted elders or those with pre-existing conditions and ruthlessly attacked those with poor metabolic health. Patients with lifestyle-related diseases like diabetes, high blood pressure, high cholesterol, and obesity were hit hardest.

Furthermore, during the third wave of COVID-19, patients often ended up on ventilators for at least three weeks, facing complications like blood clots, secondary infections, lung injuries, and delirium. Even after they survived, they didn't come out the same. They developed chronic conditions, including compromised lung function. This profoundly impacted their families, as they had to take time off work and endure immense stress and an overwhelming emotional toll. The cost of an ICU admission for a COVID-19 patient was staggering—around $50,000 per admission. But beyond the financial burden, the human cost was incalculable. Families were left grappling with the loss of normalcy and the realization that their loved ones might never return to who they were before. The effects of ICU stays were felt long after patients left the hospital, affecting their life quality, mental health, and resumption of daily activities.

A major driver of the vulnerabilities is metabolic syndrome—a cluster of conditions that include high blood sugar, high blood pressure, abnormal cholesterol levels, and excess body fat around the waist. Metabolic syndrome isn't just linked to diabetes and heart disease; it's tied to strokes, mental health issues, reproductive challenges, and even cancer. Shockingly, 87% of Americans are now considered metabolically unhealthy, and this staggering statistic underscores the urgency of the problem. The good news? Metabolic syndrome is reversible. If we lean into prevention and address the root causes, we could significantly improve our collective health and save millions from unnecessary suffering.

The realization—that we could prevent so much of the suffering—became my driving force. If we can make lifestyle changes—through diet, exercise, and stress management—we can help people avoid ever needing to see someone like me in the ICU. This isn't just about COVID-19. It's about reducing the risk of a host of diseases—stroke, cancer, heart disease, and more—by focusing on prevention. By empowering individuals with the knowledge and tools to take control of their health, we can shift the narrative from treating disease to preventing it. This shift is not just necessary; it is urgent.

> My mission now is to give people the tools
> they need to avoid the ICU.

I've spent years interviewing experts on my podcast, delving into the health and wellness space, and one thing has become abundantly clear: optimizing health doesn't have to be complicated. It can be elementary. The beauty of prevention lies in its simplicity—small, consistent changes can profoundly impact your health.

A key component of the simplicity is leveraging Pareto's Principle—the 80/20 rule. This principle suggests that 80% of your results come from 20% of your activities. In other words, we don't need to overhaul our entire lives to see significant improvements. We can achieve 80% of the health benefits by focusing on a few key lifestyle habits. This principle is a cornerstone of my approach to health: identifying the few critical changes that will yield the most significant results.

This book is about identifying the critical levers— the small changes that can make a big difference. I don't expect you to tackle all of them at once. Instead, I encourage you to choose one or two to focus on. I promise that if you stick with them, you'll immediately start seeing results. You'll feel better, move in the right direction, and ultimately take control of your health. The journey to better health is not a sprint; it's a marathon. It's about making choices today that will benefit you tomorrow and years to come.

I've heard the success stories of countless people over the past few years about how my content has helped their mom reverse type 2 diabetes, lose weight, or come off blood pressure medications. These are more than individual successes—they're life-changing transformations that often inspire families to follow suit. When one person makes a positive change, it usually creates a ripple effect, motivating others in their circle to do the same. This collective movement towards better health is what excites me the most.

> It's not just about helping one person at a time;
> it's about creating a healthier society.

This book is my attempt to guide you on that journey. I'm grateful you're here and excited to see how these strategies can help you and your loved ones lead healthier, more fulfilling lives. The power to change your life is in your hands, and it starts with the choices you make every day. I believe in the power of prevention and your ability to take control of your health.

Let's get started. Together, we can make sure that your story doesn't have to involve the ICU. Instead, it can be one of health, vitality, and longevity. Let's embark on this journey together toward a future where prevention is the norm and the ICU is the last place you'll ever need to be.

CHAPTER 2
THE POWER OF PROTEIN

"Where my protein at?"
– Dr. Kwadwo Kyeremanteng

If you've followed me on social media or listened to my podcast, you've probably heard me preach about the importance of increasing your protein intake. It's the most critical of all the steps we'll discuss regarding nutrition. In fact, if there's one thing you take away from this book, let it be the value of protein.

It's the 80/20 of the 80/20 of the 80/20—a small change that yields massive results in your overall health and well-being.

Strength in the Face of Adversity

I once took care of a patient in the ICU with a severe infection. He was in a condition that many people don't come out of the same, but there was something different about him—his dedication to strength. Despite being on life-saving medications, he insisted on keeping up his protein intake, even asking for his protein shakes while in the ICU. He maintained an impressive level of activity and barely lost any weight, which is remarkable considering that many ICU patients lose up to 1% of their lean muscle mass per day.

His outcome was nothing short of extraordinary. Where others might struggle with prolonged weakness and loss of function, he bounced back with strength. His commitment to protein intake and physical activity played a major role in his recovery. This story highlights what I tell my patients all the time: staying strong before you get sick gives you a much better shot at coming out stronger on the other side.

Why Protein Matters

I frequently see people struggling with their health, particularly with weight management, and a common thread is insufficient protein intake. Protein is an incredible macronutrient that plays a crucial role in almost every function of the body. It is responsible for:

- Building and repairing tissues

- Producing enzymes and hormones

- Supporting immune function

- Maintaining muscle mass

But that's just the beginning. Protein is essential for creating hemoglobin, the molecule in red blood cells that carries oxygen throughout your body. It plays a pivotal role in the production of neurotransmitters, which regulate mood, sleep, and cognitive functions. It also helps balance fluids, transport nutrients, and provide energy when carbohydrate and fat stores are low.

One of the biggest benefits of protein is satiety— the feeling of fullness after eating. Protein-rich foods keep you more satisfied than high-carb or high-fat foods, making you less likely to snack on unhealthy options. This makes protein a game-changer for weight management and overall health.

Protein and Metabolism

One of the reasons I believe protein is the ultimate tool for improving your health is its role in metabolism. Increasing your protein intake leads to an increase in lean muscle mass, which:

- Improves insulin sensitivity

- Enhances metabolism

- Helps regulate blood sugar levels

Muscle is metabolically active tissue, meaning it burns

calories even at rest. The more muscle you have, the higher your basal metabolic rate (BMR)—the number of calories your body burns at rest. This means that by simply eating more protein, you can naturally boost your daily calorie burn.

Protein also has a high thermic effect of food (TEF)—meaning your body burns more calories digesting protein than it does digesting carbs or fats. While fat and carbohydrates require little energy to process, protein digestion can use up to 10-15% of your total calorie intake.

How Much Protein Do You Need?

A good rule of thumb is to consume 0.7 to 1 gram of protein per pound of ideal body weight.

For example:

- A 200-pound man should aim for 140–200 grams of protein per day.

- A 150-pound woman should target 105–150 grams per day.

While this might seem like a lot, it's entirely achievable with the right approach. If you're physically active, you'll likely benefit from the higher end of this range. If you're sedentary, the lower end might be enough.

As we age, protein becomes even more important. The body becomes less efficient at using protein, making it essential for preventing muscle loss (sarcopenia). Women, especially during pregnancy and breastfeeding, may also need higher protein intake to support both their own health and their child's development.

Where to Get Your Protein

You don't need to overcomplicate it. Stick to foods you enjoy. Some of my favorite protein sources include:

- **Beef, chicken, and fish** – Nutrient-dense and packed with high-quality protein

- **Eggs** – A complete protein, loaded with essential vitamins and minerals

- **Greek yogurt** – High in protein and great for gut health

- **Cottage cheese** – A simple, high-protein snack option

- **Protein shakes** – A convenient way to boost your intake on the go

Practical Tips for Increasing Protein

I've seen firsthand that most people struggling with their weight could make significant progress just by doubling their protein intake.

- **Prioritize protein at every meal** – Start your day with eggs, have a high-protein lunch, and make sure dinner includes a lean protein source.

- **Choose smarter snacks** – Swap chips and crackers for Greek yogurt, cottage cheese, or a protein shake.

- **Ditch the fries** – When eating out, replace fries with a side salad or an extra protein portion.

- **Use a protein supplement** – If you struggle to get enough protein from food alone, a high-quality protein powder can help bridge the gap.

The Long-Term Benefits of Protein

Increasing your protein intake has profound, long-lasting effects on your health:

✓ More muscle mass → Increased strength and mobility

✓ Higher metabolism → More calories burned at rest

✓ Better insulin sensitivity → Lower risk of type 2 diabetes

✓ More stable blood sugar → Fewer cravings and more consistent energy

✓ Greater satiety → Less snacking and better weight control

Protein is not just about building muscle—it's about keeping you strong, healthy, and independent for life. The time to prioritize it s now, no matter your age or fitness level.

Reflection & Action Plan: Achieving Your Protein Goals

Take a moment to reflect on your current habits and make a plan for improvement.

1. **Identify Your Current Protein Sources**

- What are your main protein sources right now?

- Are you getting enough variety?

2. **Set Your Protein Goal**

- Based on 0.7–1 gram per pound of ideal body weight, what's your daily protein target?

- How does this compare to what you currently eat?

3. **Incorporate Protein into Each Meal**

- What are three easy ways you can increase your protein intake at breakfast, lunch, and dinner?

4. **Snack Smart**

- Can you replace a carb-heavy snack with a high-protein option?

5. Track How You Feel

- Do you feel fuller after meals?

- Do you notice fewer cravings or more energy throughout the day?

6. Make a Weekly Plan

- Plan your meals ahead of time to ensure you're hitting your protein goal.

7. Track Your Progress

- Monitor your protein intake over the next week and note any changes in energy, satiety, or overall well-being.

By prioritizing protein, you're not just making a dietary change—you're making an investment in your strength, longevity, and quality of life. Stick with it, and you'll experience the power of protein firsthand.

Worksheet: Achieving Your Protein Goals

Now that we've covered the importance of protein, it's time to think about how you can practically increase your protein intake throughout the day. Use the worksheet below to reflect on your current habits and create a plan for incorporating more protein into your diet.

1. Identify Your Current Protein Sources:

- List the main sources of protein in your diet. Are you relying heavily on one or two sources, or do you have a variety of protein-rich foods?

2. Set Your Protein Goal:

- Calculate your daily protein needs based on the recommended 0.7 to 1 gram per pound of ideal body weight. How does your current intake compare to this goal?

3. Incorporate Protein into Each Meal:

- Plan how you will include protein in each of your meals. For example, could you add eggs to your breakfast, a protein shake before lunch, and a serving of fish or chicken at dinner?

4. Snack Smart:

- Think about your snacks. Can you replace a carbohydrate-heavy snack with a protein-rich one? For example, swap chips for Greek yogurt or a handful of nuts.

5. Reflect on How You Feel Post-Meal:

- Pay attention to how you feel after meals when you increase your protein intake. Are you more satisfied? Do you notice fewer cravings? How is your energy level throughout the day?

6. Make a Weekly Plan:

∘ Create a weekly meal plan that prioritizes protein at every meal. Consider batch cooking or prepping your protein sources in advance to make it easier to stay on track.

Monday:

Tuesday:

Wednesday:

Thursday:

Friday:

Saturday:

Sunday:

7. Track Your Progress:

By incorporating more protein into your daily routine, you'll likely find that you feel fuller, more satisfied, and more energetic—key factors in achieving and maintaining optimal health. Stick with it, and you'll be well on your way to reaping the benefits of this powerful macronutrient.

CHAPTER 3
THE POWER OF FASTING

"Metabolic health is your greatest defense."
– Dr. Kwadwo Kyeremanteng

Dr. Tom Psarras: Taking Control of Health

One of my favorite stories from the pandemic is that of my colleague, Dr. Tom Psarras. As an ICU doctor, he saw firsthand the devastating impact of poor metabolic health on COVID-19 outcomes. Patients with obesity, type 2 diabetes, and metabolic syndrome were at much higher risk of severe complications, ICU admissions, and even death. Seeing this direct link, Dr. Psarras was motivated to take action—on himself.

Rather than just treating patients, he took control of his own health by incorporating intermittent fasting and a low-carb diet to improve his metabolic status. Within a few months, he was down 30 pounds, had significantly improved his insulin sensitivity, and reduced his risk of not just severe COVID, but also heart disease, stroke, cancer, and even mood disorders.

It was truly inspirational to watch him go through this transformation. He didn't just accept the status quo— he made real, lasting changes. His story is a powerful reminder that we have more control over our health than we often believe.

Why Fasting Works

Fasting isn't just about weight loss. It's about metabolic health. When you fast, several powerful changes occur in your body:

- Lower insulin levels → Makes it easier to burn fat for energy.

- Increased autophagy → The body's natural process of cleaning out damaged cells and regenerating new ones.

- Better blood sugar control → Helps prevent and even reverse insulin resistance.

- Reduced inflammation → Chronic inflammation is linked to heart disease, cancer, and autoimmune conditions.

Most of us eat too often—three meals a day plus snacks—and never allow our body to tap into stored fat for energy. Fasting is one of the simplest ways to reset your metabolism and improve long-term health.

The Benefits of Intermittent Fasting

1. Weight Loss & Fat Burning

- Fasting forces your body to use stored fat for energy.

- It also increases levels of human growth hormone (HGH), which helps preserve muscle while burning fat.

2. Improved Insulin Sensitivity

- Chronically high insulin is a major driver of metabolic disease.

- Fasting helps lower insulin levels, reducing the risk of type 2 diabetes.

3. Reduced Risk of Chronic Disease

- Studies show fasting can lower blood pressure, cholesterol, and inflammation—key risk factors for heart disease and stroke.

- It has also been linked to reduced cancer risk, possibly due to its effects on cellular repair and autophagy.

4. Better Brain Function

- Fasting increases levels of BDNF (Brain-Derived Neurotrophic Factor), which supports brain health and may lower the risk of Alzheimer's and Parkinson's disease.

- Many people report better focus, mental clarity, and even improved mood when fasting.

How to Get Started with Fasting

If you're new to fasting, start slow. You don't need to jump into extreme fasting protocols—small changes can make a big difference.

- **16:8 Method** → Fast for 16 hours and eat within an 8-hour window (e.g., noon to 8 PM).

- **20:4 Method** (OMAD - One Meal a Day) → A shorter eating window, often used for weight loss.

- **5:2 Method** → Eat normally 5 days a week and consume fewer calories (500-600) on 2 non-consecutive days.

The key is consistency. Like Dr. Psarras, you may be surprised at how quickly your body adapts and how much better you feel.

Common Concerns About Fasting

1. "Won't I lose muscle?"

- No. Fasting preserves muscle by increasing HGH and improving fat oxidation.

- Resistance training while fasting can further protect muscle mass.

2. "Will I feel weak or lightheaded?"

- If you feel weak, it may be due to electrolyte imbalances (low sodium, magnesium, or potassium).

- Drink salt water or bone broth to help.

3. "Is fasting safe for women?"

- Yes, but women may need to adjust fasting lengths based on menstrual cycles and energy levels.

- Start with 12-14 hours of fasting and increase gradually.

4. "Can I drink coffee or tea?"

- Yes! Black coffee, tea, and water are fine during fasting periods.

  During fasting periods, black coffee, tea, and water are totally fine. In general, as a rule of thumb, consuming less than 50 calories is unlikely to break your fast—so a splash of milk or a bit of cream in your coffee or tea is probably okay. Just keep it minimal and avoid added sugars to stay within that fasting-safe zone.

Practical Tips for Successful Fasting

✓ Stay hydrated – Drink plenty of water, black coffee, or herbal tea.

✓ Prioritize protein – When breaking your fast, eat high-protein, nutrient-dense foods.

✓ Get enough electrolytes – Salt, magnesium, and potassium can help avoid fatigue and headaches.

✓ Listen to your body – If you feel unwell, adjust your fasting window or increase protein intake.

✓ Be consistent – The benefits of fasting compound over time. Stick with it!

The Long-Term Benefits of Fasting

By incorporating fasting into your routine, you're not just losing weight—you're improving your metabolic health, reducing disease risk, and increasing longevity.

✓ Lower risk of type 2 diabetes

✓ Improved heart health

✓ Better brain function & mood stability

✓ Increased fat-burning & better body composition

Dr. Psarras's story proves that metabolic health is in your hands. He didn't wait for a diagnosis—he took action. And you can too.

Reflection & Action Plan: Is Fasting Right for You?

Take a few minutes to reflect on your current eating habits and consider whether fasting could be a useful tool for you.

- Do you think fasting is for you? Why or why not?

- What are your main concerns about trying fasting?

- If you've tried fasting before, how did it make you feel?

- What are some barriers that might make fasting challenging for you?

- What other strategies might be useful for improving your metabolic health?

- Could you commit to a small fasting window (12-14 hours) to start?

By reflecting on these questions, you can decide whether fasting is a strategy worth incorporating into your lifestyle. Remember, small, sustainable changes lead to lasting results.

If Dr. Psarras could transform his metabolic health in a matter of months, so can you. Take control of your health—it's one of the best investments you'll ever make.

Conclusion

Intermittent fasting is one of the most efficient ways to reset your metabolism, support weight management, and enhance overall health. It's not just about when you eat; it's about giving your body the space to function optimally. Whether you're new to fasting or looking to refine your practice, these tips and strategies will help you effectively incorporate fasting into your life.

Remember, health is a journey, not a sprint. Start small, stay consistent, and watch your body transform.

Worksheet: Create Your Fasting Plan

Use this worksheet to develop a fasting strategy that suits your needs:

1. Choose Your Fasting Method:

- 12-Hour Fast

- 16/8 Method

- 24-Hour Fast

- 5:2 Diet

- Other: _____

2. Set Your Goals:

- Why are you fasting? (e.g., weight loss, better focus, improved metabolism)

  _____

3. Plan Your Meals:

- First meal after fasting: _____

- Favorite fasting-friendly snacks: _____

4. Track Your Progress:

- Date: _____

- Fasting Duration: _____

- How I Felt: _____

5. Troubleshooting:

- What challenges did you face today?

  _____

- What can you adjust tomorrow?

  _____

CHAPTER 4
AVOID PROCESSED FOODS—
FUEL YOUR BODY WITH WHOLE
FOODS

"The middle of the grocery store? Straight-up medieval!"
– Dr. Kwadwo Kyeremanteng

The Power of Elimination

I had a good friend who was extremely overweight. She had clear signs of metabolic syndrome—high blood sugar, high blood pressure, and excess body fat around the waist. But beyond that, she was also struggling with depression. She felt trapped in her own body, unsure of how to break the cycle.

One day, she made one simple change—she cut out pop. At the time, she was drinking anywhere from 4 to 6 cans of regular Coke per day. She first switched to diet soda, then eventually quit altogether. That single decision helped her lose 10% of her body weight—about 30 pounds.

But the most beautiful part? That small win gave her confidence. It started her journey toward better health. Today, she still faces challenges, but she's in a much better place than she was years ago. Her story proves that eliminating just one processed food can have a massive impact on metabolic health.

The Problem with Processed Foods

We live in a world where processed foods dominate our diets. They're everywhere—grocery store aisles, restaurant menus, vending machines. They're cheap, convenient, and engineered to be addictive. But they come at a serious cost to our health.

Processed foods are packed with:

✓ Added sugars → Spikes blood sugar, increases fat storage, and contributes to insulin resistance.

✓ Unhealthy fats → Trans fats and seed oils promote inflammation and heart disease.

✓ Artificial additives → Preservatives, sweeteners, and flavor enhancers disrupt gut health and brain function.

✓ Excessive sodium → Can contribute to high blood pressure and fluid retention.

Switching to whole, minimally processed foods is one of the most powerful changes you can make to improve your health.

What Are Processed Foods?

Not all processing is bad. Some foods are minimally processed for convenience or safety, while others are ultra-processed and should be minimized or avoided.

- Minimally Processed Foods → Slightly altered but still nutrient-dense (e.g., frozen vegetables, canned beans, plain yogurt).

- Ultra-Processed Foods → Heavily altered with additives, sugars, and preservatives (e.g., soda, chips, fast food, sugary cereals).

- The goal isn't perfection—it's reducing your intake of ultra-processed foods while prioritizing whole, nutrient-dense options.

Why Processed Foods Are Harmful

Ultra-processed foods strip away nutrients and replace them with harmful ingredients. Here's why they should be minimized:

1. They're Nutrient-Poor

- Processing removes fiber, vitamins, and minerals.

- Leaves behind empty calories that don't fuel your body.

2. **They Spike Blood Sugar & Insulin**

- High in added sugars → Causes energy crashes and increased fat storage.

- Leads to insulin resistance, a major risk factor for diabetes and metabolic disease.

3. **They Promote Overeating**

- Designed for "hyper-palatability" → Makes you crave more food.

- You eat more without feeling full, leading to weight gain.

4. **They Increase Inflammation**

- Trans fats and seed oils contribute to chronic inflammation.

- Linked to heart disease, Alzheimer's, and autoimmune conditions.

5. **They Impact Mood & Mental Health**

- Processed foods can disrupt gut health, affecting dopamine and serotonin levels.

- High sugar intake is linked to increased risk of depression and anxiety.

The Benefits of Whole Foods

Switching to whole foods can transform your health in just a few months. Some key benefits:

✓ Steady Energy Levels → No more sugar crashes.

✓ Better Digestion → Fiber supports gut health.

✓ Reduced Inflammation → Supports heart health & immune function.

✓ Easier Weight Management → Whole foods are naturally filling.

✓ Stronger Metabolic Health → Lower blood sugar & insulin resistance.

The key to long-term health isn't a restrictive diet—it's simply eating more whole, nutrient-dense foods.

How to Transition Away from Processed Foods

Making this shift doesn't have to be overwhelming. Small, consistent changes can lead to big results.

1. Shop the Perimeter

- Fresh fruits, vegetables, meat, eggs, dairy, and whole grains are on the outer edges of the grocery store.

- Avoid the middle aisles filled with ultra-processed snacks and packaged foods.

2. Read Labels

- Choose foods with 5 ingredients or fewer.

- Avoid added sugars, hydrogenated oils, and artificial preservatives.

3. Cook at Home

- Preparing your own meals gives you full control over ingredients.

- Meal prep doesn't have to be complicated—start with simple, whole-food meals.

4. Replace, Don't Eliminate

- Instead of cutting out foods entirely, swap them for healthier alternatives:

Processed Food	Whole Food Alternative
Sugary cereal	Oatmeal with fresh fruit
White bread	Sprouted or whole-grain bread
Soda	Sparkling water with lemon
Chips	Roasted nuts or air-popped popcorn
Packaged frozen meals	Home-cooked meals or leftovers

5. Prioritize Protein & Fiber

- Lean proteins (chicken, fish, eggs, tofu) keep you full.

- Fiber-rich foods (vegetables, beans, whole grains) support gut health.

6. Plan Your Meals

- Having a plan prevents impulse purchases of processed foods.

- Meal prepping saves time and money.

7. Allow for Flexibility

- Perfection isn't the goal. It's okay to have treats occasionally—just don't make them the foundation of your diet.

Common Barriers & How to Overcome Them

✓ "I don't have time to cook." → Try batch cooking or using a slow cooker.

✓ "Healthy food is expensive." → Buy in bulk, choose frozen produce, and shop seasonally.

✓ "I crave processed foods." → Replace them with satisfying whole-food snacks.

✓ "I eat out often." → Choose restaurants with whole-food options and avoid sugary drinks.

Reflection & Action Plan: Reducing Processed Foods

Take a few minutes to reflect on your current diet and set a plan for improvement.

- What processed foods do you eat most often?

- What's one processed food you could eliminate this week?

- What whole-food alternatives could you try?

- How do you feel after eating whole foods vs. processed foods?

- What's one action step you'll take to reduce processed foods this week?

Final Thoughts: Small Changes, Big Impact

My friend's story proves that one small change can spark an entire health transformation. Eliminating processed foods isn't about perfection—it's about progress.

✓ Start with one swap (cut out soda, add more protein, cook at home).

✓ Notice how you feel—better energy, fewer cravings, improved mood.

✓ Keep building momentum—small wins lead to big results.

Your health is in your hands. Make the choice today to fuel your body with the nutrients it deserves.

Conclusion

> Reducing processed foods isn't about perfection—
> it's about making progress.

Every step toward incorporating whole foods into your diet improves your health, energy, and overall quality of life. Small, consistent changes add up to significant results, so start where you are and celebrate every win along the way.

Take charge of your health today—your body will thank you!

Worksheet: Your Whole Foods Plan

Use this worksheet to kickstart your journey:

1. **Assess Your Current Diet**

   List three processed foods you eat most often:

   _____

2. **Identify Whole Food Swaps**

   Write healthier alternatives: _____

3. **Plan One Whole-Food Meal**

   Choose a meal you can prepare: _____

4. **Set a Weekly Goal**

   What's one action you'll take this week to reduce processed foods?

5. **Track Your Progress**

   Note how you feel after each meal:

   - Meal 1: _____
   - Meal 2: _____

CHAPTER 5
LIFT WEIGHTS—BUILDING STRENGTH FOR LIFELONG HEALTH

"Strength does not come from winning. Your struggles develop your strengths. When you go through hardships and decide not to surrender, that is strength."
— Arnold Schwarzenegger

Lifting weights is one of the most transformative habits you can adopt when it comes to exercise. It's not just for bodybuilders or athletes—resistance training is for everyone, regardless of age or fitness level. Incorporating weightlifting into your routine builds strength, supports metabolic health, and helps prevent various chronic conditions. In fact, resistance training is so powerful that it's often called the "fountain of youth" in the health and fitness world.

Lifting weights isn't just about aesthetics or building muscle for appearance's sake. It's about enhancing your overall functionality, protecting your body from injury, and ensuring you can maintain independence and vitality as you age.

A Real-Life Reminder: Strength Saved His Life

I'll never forget a patient I once cared for—a man in his mid-70s who suffered a cardiac arrest. Now, in my world, when someone in their 70s experiences a cardiac arrest—essentially dying for a period of time—the prognosis is often grim. Most don't survive. Those who do frequently end up so deconditioned they require long-term care or transition to a nursing home.

But this man was different.

Why? Because he had what I like to call body armor— a solid foundation of strength built through years of consistency. He went to the gym five days a week. That dedication made all the difference. Even while on a ventilator, he was able to walk. Let me say that again— this man walked while on a ventilator. That kind of resilience is extremely rare and speaks volumes about the protective power of muscle mass and physical conditioning.

His physical strength wasn't the only factor—he also had the mental fortitude that comes from years of discipline. Anyone who's stayed committed to a training routine, especially when motivation is low, knows how that grit carries over into other areas of life. And in the ICU, that grit can be the difference between giving up and fighting through.

Today, he's at home, spending time with his grandkids. And that wouldn't have been possible without the years he invested in his health.

That's the power of lifting weights. That's the power of strength.

For those who aren't ready to lift heavy weights or don't have access to a gym, bodyweight exercises and high-intensity interval training (HIIT) provide excellent alternatives that deliver remarkable benefits.

The Benefits of Resistance Training

Weightlifting offers a wide range of physical and mental health benefits that go far beyond muscle growth:

1. Builds Lean Muscle Mass:

Muscle mass naturally declines with age, due to a condition known as sarcopenia. Resistance training combats this decline, ensuring you maintain strength and mobility as you age.

2. Boosts Metabolic Rate:

Muscle tissue burns more calories at rest than fat tissue. The more muscle you have, the higher your basal metabolic rate (BMR), meaning you'll burn more calories throughout the day—even when you're not exercising.

3. Improves Insulin Sensitivity:

One of the most profound benefits of resistance training is its ability to improve insulin sensitivity. Strength training increases your muscles' ability to absorb glucose from the bloodstream and use it for energy, which lowers blood sugar leve s. This makes weightlifting and bodyweight exercises powerful tools for preventing and even reversing type 2 diabetes.

4. Strengthens Bones and Joints:

Weight-bearing exercises stimulate bone growth and increase its density to reduce osteoporosis risk. Strengthening the muscles around your joints also decreases the likelihood of injury.

5. Enhances Physical Resilience:

A strong body is better equipped to handle physical challenges like carrying groceries and recovering from illness or injury.

6. Supports Mental Health:

Resistance training has been shown to reduce depression and anxiety symptoms, improve mood, and boost self-confidence.

7. Prevents Frailty:

As an ICU doctor, I've seen how frailty contributes to poor patient outcomes. Weightlifting or consistent bodyweight exercises can help you maintain strength and mobility, reducing your risk of falls and hospitalizations later in life.

Exercise Snacks—Small Efforts, Big Impact

One of the easiest ways to integrate strength training into your day is through **exercise snacks**—short bursts of activity that can be done throughout the day. These mini-workouts are perfect for people with busy schedules or those looking to add more movement to their routines.

Here are some examples of exercise snacks:

- **Squats:** Perform 10–20 air squats during commercial breaks or while waiting for your coffee to brew. Squats engage your glutes, quads, and core to improve strength and mobility.

- **Push-Ups:** Drop down for 5–15 push-ups in between tasks. Push-ups strengthen your chest, shoulders, and triceps while engaging your core.

- **Burpees:** Knock out a quick set of 5–10 burpees for a full-body workout that gets your heart rate up.

- **Planks:** Hold a plank for 30–60 seconds to build core stability and overall strength.

Exercise snacks improve your physical health and boost your mood and energy levels throughout the day. These brief movements can add up, making a significant difference in your overall fitness.

HIIT: Maximizing Time and Effort

For those who want to pack a lot in a short time, **high-intensity interval training (HIIT)** is a great option. It involves alternating between bursts of intense activity and short recovery periods, making it a time-efficient way to improve cardiovascular fitness, burn calories, and build strength.

Example of HIIT Workouts:

1. **Tabata Kettlebell Swings:**

   Perform kettlebell swings for 20 seconds at maximum effort, followed by 10 seconds of rest. Repeat for 8 rounds (a total of 4 minutes). For a super-quick workout, you can complete 1–2 Tabata rounds.

2. Bodyweight Circuit:

- 30 seconds of jump squats

- 30 seconds of mountain climbers

- 30 seconds of burpees

- 30 seconds of rest

  Repeat for 3–4 rounds.

HIIT workouts provide an efficient way to incorporate cardio and strength training into your routine, especially if you're pressed for time.

Bodyweight Workout Routine

For those who don't have access to gym equipment, a bodyweight workout can be an excellent alternative. Here's a simple routine that targets your entire body:

1. Bodyweight Squats: 3 sets of 15 reps

- Strengthens your glutes, quads, and hamstrings.

2. Push-Ups: 3 sets of 10–15 reps (modify to knee push-ups if needed)

- Builds upper-body strength, targeting the chest, shoulders, and triceps.

3. **Lunges (Each Leg): 3 sets of 10 reps per leg**

  ◦ Improves balance and strengthens the lower body.

4. **Plank Hold: 3 rounds of 30 seconds**

  ◦ Builds core stability and improves posture.

5. **Glute Bridges: 3 sets of 12–15 reps**

  ◦ Strengthens the glutes and lower back.

6. **Mountain Climbers: 3 rounds of 30 seconds**

  ◦ A dynamic exercise that targets the core and gets your heart rate up.

This workout requires no equipment and can be done in as little as 15–20 minutes. It's perfect for beginners or anyone looking to stay active without a gym.

Why Compound Lifts Are My Favorite

Compound lifts are a fantastic addition if you're ready to advance beyond bodyweight exercises. These exercises work multiple muscle groups simultaneously, offering an efficient and effective way to build strength.

Here are reasons why compound lifts are so valuable:

1. **Efficient Workouts:**

   Compound movements target multiple areas at once, saving time while maximizing results. For example, a deadlift engages your hamstrings, glutes, core, and lower back.

2. **Build Functional Strength:**

   These exercises mimic real-life movements, such as lifting, pushing, and pulling, enhancing your strength for daily activities.

3. **Stimulate Hormone Production:**

   Compound lifts stimulate the release of anabolic hormones like testosterone and growth hormone, which promote muscle growth and overall health.

4. **Burn More Calories:**

   Because compound lifts recruit large muscle groups, they have a high caloric demand, making them ideal for weight loss and metabolic health.

5. **Improve Insulin Sensitivity:**

   Compound lifts are particularly effective at enhancing insulin sensitivity, helping prevent or manage type 2 diabetes.

Practical Weightlifting Plan

Here's a beginner-friendly weightlifting plan to help you get started:

1. **Squats (Bodyweight or Weighted):** 3 sets of 10–12 reps

2. **Push-Ups or Bench Press:** 3 sets of 10–12 reps

3. **Dumbbell Rows (Per Arm):** 3 sets of 10 reps

4. **Deadlifts (If Available):** 3 sets of 10 reps

5. **Plank Hold:** 3 rounds of 30 seconds

You can integrate HIIT sessions or exercise snacks into your week for added intensity.

My Personal Experience

I've seen the benefits of resistance training both personally and professionally. Patients who incorporate weightlifting often report feeling stronger and experiencing fewer aches and pains, improved energy levels, and better metabolic health.

I love incorporating **compound lifts** like squats and deadlifts into my routine—they offer unmatched efficiency and results. I rely on exercise snacks and HIIT sessions on busy days to stay active, even if I only have a few minutes to spare.

One of my favorite examples is a patient who started with just bodyweight exercises during commercial breaks. Within weeks, they noticed improved energy, better mood, and increased strength, which motivated them to progress to more structured workouts. These small changes can lead to big results.

Conclusion

Lifting weights, performing bodyweight exercises, and incorporating HIIT are powerful tools for improving your health and longevity. Whether you're using traditional gym equipment, doing bodyweight circuits, or squeezing in exercise snacks throughout the day, the key is consistency.

By committing to strength training, you'll feel stronger and set the foundation for a healthier, more vibrant future.

Worksheet: Building Strength for Lifelong Health

1. Reflection Questions:

- Why is strength training important for overall health and longevity?

- What are some misconceptions you've had (or heard) about lifting weights?

- Have you ever incorporated strength training into your routine? If so, what has worked well for you? If not, what has held you back?

2. Understanding the Benefits:

∘ Match each benefit of strength training with its correct explanation:

A. Improved Metabolism	1. _____ Strength training increases bone density, lowering the risk of osteoporosis.
B. Stronger Bones	2. _____ Muscle tissue burns more calories than fat, helping with weight management.
C. Better Mental Health	3. _____ Lifting weights can reduce symptoms of anxiety and depression.
D. Reduced Risk of Chronic Disease	4. _____ Strength allows you to perform daily activities more easily (e.g., carrying groceries, climbing stairs).
E. Improved Daily Function	5. _____ Regular resistance training lowers the risk of conditions like heart disease and diabetes.

3. Personal Strength Training Plan:

- What are your current strength levels? (e.g., beginner, intermediate, advanced)

- What type of strength training interests you the most? (e.g., bodyweight exercises, free weights, machines, resistance bands)

- How many days per week can you realistically commit to strength training?

- What obstacles might get in your way, and how can you overcome them?

4. Action Steps:

Create a simple strength training plan for the next week. Choose at least three exercises from the list below and write down when you'll do them.

Exercise Options:

- Squats

- Push-ups

- Deadlifts

- Lunges

- Rows

- Planks

My Plan:

- Day 1: _____
- Day 2: _____
- Day 3: _____

5. Tracking Progress:

Over the next four weeks, track your strength training sessions. What changes do you notice in your energy, strength, or overall well-being?

Date	Workout completed	How I Felt After

CHAPTER 6
INCREASE YOUR STEPS—
A SIMPLE PATH TO BETTER
HEALTH

"Walking is man's best medicine."
— Hippocrates

The Power of Walking: A Tribute to My Dad

Writing this chapter brought up a lot of emotions because when I think about walking, I think about my dad. He's no longer with us, but if there was one thing he was known for, it was walking.

My dad wasn't a fitness fanatic. In fact, looking back, I realize he was probably 30 pounds overweight and likely had metabolic syndrome. But at some point in his life, something clicked. I don't know what sparked it, but he decided to take control of his health, and walking was one of the main ways he did it.

And when I say walking, I mean walking everywhere. He walked for hours. It became part of his identity. People would see him all over the city and come up to me and say, "I saw your dad walking in this part of town today." It was just who he was.

As a kid, I didn't get it. I used to watch him and think, "Why does he do this?" Walking is so boring.

But now, in my middle age, I get it. I love it. The fresh air, the ability to listen to a book, enjoy music, or have a deep conversation with a friend—walking is so much more than just movement. It's therapy. It's freedom. It's a simple, powerful way to take control of your health.

And when I think of the true benefits of walking—for physical health, mental well-being, longevity, and even sleep—I can't help but picture my dad, moving through the streets of Edmonton with his determined pace, living his best life.

Why Walking Matters

Walking might seem too simple to be effective, but research shows it's one of the most beneficial forms of physical activity.

✓ Improves Cardiovascular Health → Strengthens the heart, lowers blood pressure, and reduces the risk of heart disease.

✓ Supports Weight Management → Burns calories and prevents weight gain.

✓ Enhances Metabolic Health → Walking after meals helps stabilize blood sugar levels and reduces insulin resistance.

✓ Boosts Mental Health → Reduces stress, anxiety, and depression while improving mood and focus.

✓ Promotes Longevity → Higher daily step counts are linked to longer life expectancy.

✓ Improves Sleep Quality → Walking during the day helps regulate sleep cycles.

The best part? It's accessible to almost everyone. No gym. No equipment. No cost.

How Many Steps Do You Need?

The 10,000-step goal is widely promoted, but research shows you don't need that many to see real benefits.

General Guidelines:

- Sedentary (<5,000 steps/day) → Add 1,000–2,000 steps daily.

- Moderately Active (5,000–7,000 steps/day) → Aim for 7,000–8,000 steps daily.

- Highly Active (>8,000 steps/day) → Maintain your activity or increase intensity.

Even just 7,000 steps a day can significantly lower your risk of chronic disease and early death.

How to Increase Your Daily Steps

You don't have to schedule extra workouts—just find simple ways to add movement to your day.

- ✓ Take Walking Breaks → Set a timer to walk for 5 minutes every hour.

- ✓ Use Walking as Transportation → Walk instead of driving for short trips.

- ✓ Schedule Walking Meetings → Take work calls or meetings on the move.

- ✓ Walk After Meals → A 10–15 minute walk after meals can stabilize blood sugar.

- ✓ Make It Social → Walk with a friend or family member.

- ✓ Explore New Routes → Keep it interesting by changing your walking locations.

- ✓ Track Your Steps → Use a fitness tracker or phone app to stay motivated.

- ✓ Pair Walking with Other Activities → Listen to music, podcasts, or audiobooks.

Walking isn't something extra—it's a habit you can seamlessly integrate into your daily life.

The Role of Walking in Metabolic Health

One of the most powerful things about walking is its impact on metabolic health.

1. Reduces Insulin Resistance → Helps muscles absorb glucose, lowering blood sugar.

2. Boosts Caloric Expenditure → Burns energy without adding stress to the body.

3. Improves Post-Meal Blood Sugar → Short walks after meals significantly reduce blood sugar spikes.

This is why walking is so effective for preventing and managing type 2 diabetes. It's low impact, easy to do, and incredibly powerful.

My Personal Experience

Walking has been one of the most consistent forms of exercise in my life.

As a busy professional and father, I don't always have time for long gym sessions, but I can always find time to walk. Whether it's a quick walk after meals or a walking meeting at work, I make it a priority.

One of my patients had high blood sugar and low energy. I encouraged them to start walking for just 15 minutes after meals and gradually increase their daily steps. Within weeks, they saw dramatic improvements in their glucose levels, energy, and mood.

Walking is transformative,
and it doesn't take much to see real results.

Key Takeaways

✓ Walking is one of the most effective ways to improve your health.

✓ Even 7,000 steps a day can reduce disease risk and increase longevity.

✓ You don't need a gym—just move more throughout the day.

✓ Walking after meals is one of the best habits for blood sugar control.

✓ Pair walking with other activities (music, audiobooks, social time) to stay engaged.

Reflection & Action Plan: Increasing Your Steps

1. How many steps do you currently take per day?

2. What's a realistic step goal for next week?

3. List three ways you can add more steps to your routine.

4. How does walking make you feel physically and mentally?

Tips for Staying Consistent

✓ Make It Convenient → Walk during natural breaks in your day.

✓ Set Reminders → Use alarms or phone notifications.

✓ Reward Yourself → Celebrate milestones, like hitting 5,000 steps for the first time.

✓ Stay Flexible → If you miss a day, don't stress. Just keep moving forward.

Final Thoughts: Every Step Counts

Walking is one of the simplest yet most powerful ways to improve your health.

It's not about perfection—it's about small, consistent efforts that add up over time. Whether you start with 5,000 steps or 10 minutes of walking after meals, you're making a choice to invest in your long-term health.

When I think of what walking truly represents, I picture my dad, power-walking through the streets of Edmonton, fully present in his body.

I hope this chapter inspires you to take those steps—not just for your health, but for the mental clarity, longevity, and simple joy that walking can bring.

So, lace up your shoes, take a deep breath, and start moving. Every step counts.

Conclusion

Walking is one of the simplest yet most effective ways to improve your health and well-being. Increasing your daily steps can boost your cardiovascular health, support weight management, and enhance your metabolic profile without you needing expensive equipment or gym memberships. The best part? Walking is accessible to nearly everyone and can be tailored to fit your lifestyle.

Remember, every step counts. Start small, stay consistent, and celebrate your progress along the way. With walking as part of your routine, you're taking a powerful step toward a healthier, more active life.

Worksheet: Your Step-Boosting Plan

Use this worksheet to create a plan for increasing your daily steps:

1. Assess Your Current Steps:

- How many steps do you typically take in a day?

_____

2. Set a Step Goal:

- What's your target for next week?

_____

3. Identify Opportunities for Walking:

- List three ways you can add more steps to your day (e.g., walking breaks, parking farther away, walking after meals):

_____

4. Track Your Progress:

- Use the following space to log your steps for the week:

Day 1: _____

Day 2: _____

Day 3: _____

5. Reflect on Your Experience:

- How did you feel after increasing your steps?

_____

CHAPTER 7
PRACTICE YOGA—STRENGTHEN YOUR BODY AND CALM YOUR MIND

"Yoga is the journey of the self, through the self, to the self."
— The Bhagavad Gita

The Power of Yoga: Inspired by My Wife

When I think of yoga, I think of my wife, Catherine Kyeremanteng. She's a neuropsychologist, and her passion for yoga and mindfulness has been truly inspiring.

She doesn't just practice yoga for herself—she integrates it into her work, using it to help patients recover from brain injuries like concussions and traumatic brain injuries (TBI). She's shown me firsthand how yoga isn't just about flexibility or relaxation—it's about healing, resilience, and the mind-body connection.

Seeing the impact she's had—not only on her patients but also on the people around her—has been eye-opening. She's an advocate for movement and mindfulness, and I've learned so much from her.

Personally, yoga has been a godsend for me. I've had minor injuries—back pain, hip issues—and yoga has helped me recover and stay mobile. But beyond the physical benefits, I've realized that yoga has this incredible ability to ground you, to bring you back into balance.

And in a world that's constantly moving at full speed, we all need that.

So, Catherine—if by some chance you read this (which I doubt you will)—love you, and thank you for everything.

Why Yoga Matters

Yoga isn't just about stretching or posing on a mat—it's a holistic practice that benefits both your body and mind.

- ✓ Improves Flexibility & Mobility → Enhances joint health, reduces stiffness, and prevents injury.

- ✓ Builds Strength → Engages multiple muscle groups, improving functional strength.

✓ Enhances Balance → Reduces the risk of falls and improves coordination.

✓ Reduces Stress & Anxiety → Breathing techniques calm the nervous system and lower stress hormones.

✓ Supports Mental Health → Yoga is linked to reduced symptoms of depression and anxiety.

✓ Improves Sleep Qua ty → Helps regulate your body's stress response and promotes relaxation.

✓ Boosts Cardiovascular Health → Certain styles, like Vinyasa o Power Yoga, elevate heart rate and improve endurance.

✓ Encourages Mind-Body Awareness → Helps you tune into your body's neecs, leading to better overall health.

Yoga isn't just about physical fitness—it's about finding balance, both inside and out.

Types of Yoga

There are many different styles of yoga, depending on your goals:

✓ Hatha Yoga → Great for beginners; focuses on basic poses and breathing.

✓ Vinyasa Yoga → A more dynamic, flowing style that links breath to movement.

✓ Ashtanga Yoga → A challenging, structured sequence of poses best for those seeking intensity.

✓ Yin Yoga → Slower, deep stretching for improved flexibility and relaxation.

✓ Restorative Yoga → Uses props (bolsters, blankets) for deep relaxation and stress relief.

✓ Power Yoga → A fitness-based style focused on strength and endurance.

✓ Chair Yoga → A modified version of yoga for people with mobility issues.

There's a yoga style for everyone, whether you want to de-stress, build strength, or improve flexibility.

Getting Started with Yoga

If you're new to yoga, here's how to ease into it:

✓ Start Slow → Try beginner-friendly classes like Hatha or Restorative Yoga.

✓ Be Consistent → Even 10 minutes a day can make a difference.

✓ Focus on Breath → Breathing deeply helps calm your nervous system.

✓ Listen to Your Body → Modify poses as needed—no need to push into pain.

✓ Create a Yoga Space → A quiet, clutter-free area can help you establish a routine.

✓ Use Props → Blocks, straps, and bolsters make poses more accessible.

✓ Pair Yoga with Other Workouts → It complements weightlifting, walking, or HIIT.

Yoga isn't about perfection—it's about practice.

A Simple Yoga Flow for Beginners

Here's a quick 10-minute routine to get you started:

1. **Child's Pose (Balasana) → 1–2 minutes**

   ◦ Relaxes your back, shoulders, and hips.

2. **Cat-Cow Stretch → 1 minute**

   ◦ Warms up the spine and improves mobility.

3. **Downward Dog → 1 minute**

   ◦ Stretches hamstrings, calves, and spine.

4. **Warrior I → 30 seconds per side**

   ◦ Builds leg and core strength.

5. **Tree Pose → 30 seconds per side**
   ◦ Improves balance and coordination.

6. **Seated Forward Fold → 1–2 minutes**

- ◦ Releases tension in the lower back and hamstrings.

7. **Legs-Up-the-Wall Pose → 2 minutes**

- Encourages circulation and relaxation.

This simple flow is perfect for beginners—gentle but effective.

Key Takeaways

✓ Yoga improves strength, flexibility, and mental clarity.

✓ It reduces stress and enhances overall well-being.

✓ You don't need to be flexible to start—just begin.

✓ Breathing and mindfulness are just as important as the poses.

✓ Consistency matters more than intensity.

Yoga is a practice—not a performance.

Reflection & Action Plan: Starting Your Yoga Journey

- What interests you most about yoga? (Stress relief, flexibility, strength?)

- Which type of yoga do you want to try?

- How many times a week can you realistically practice?

- How do you feel after trying yoga?

Jot down your answers and set a simple goal—maybe one session this week.

My Personal Experience

Yoga has been life-changing for me, both personally and professionally.

As an ICU doctor, the stress of work can be overwhelming. Yoga gives me a way to reset, breathe, and stay grounded.

And I've seen yoga change lives.

I worked with a woman in her 60s who had chronic joint pain and anxiety. She started with chair yoga and gradually progressed to more dynamic poses. Over time, she regained mobility, reduced her stress, and felt more in control of her health.

That's the power of yoga.

Tips for Staying Consistent

✓ Make it easy → Pick a time/place that fits your routine.

✓ Set reminders → Schedule yoga sessions like an appointment.

✓ Start small → Even 5–10 minutes counts.

✓ Track progress → Write down how you feel after each session.

✓ Be patient → Yoga is a journey, not a race.

Final Thoughts: Yoga as a Lifelong Practice

Yoga isn't just about exercise—it's about showing up for yourself.

> It's about strengthening your body, calming your mind, and creating balance in a chaotic world.

And if you're still hesitant, just remember: you don't need to be flexible, fit, or experienced to start. You just need willingness and consistency.

Whether you practice for stress relief, strength, mobility, or mental clarity, yoga will change your life.

So roll out your mat, take a deep breath, and begin. You won't regret it.

Conclusion

Yoga is more than just an exercise—it's a practice that nurtures your body, mind, and spirit. Incorporating yoga into your routine can help you build strength, improve flexibility, and reduce stress while fostering a deeper connection with yourself. Whether you spend 10 minutes or an hour on the mat, the benefits of yoga will extend far beyond the practice itself.

Remember, yoga is a journey, not a destination. Start where you are, be patient, and enjoy the transformation process.

Worksheet: Your Yoga Practice Plan

Use this worksheet to create a personalized yoga routine:

1. Set Your Goals:

- Why do you want to practice yoga? (e.g., reduce stress, improve flexibility, build strength)

_____

2. Choose a Style:

- Which type of yoga appeals to you? (e.g., Hatha, Vinyasa, Yin)

_____

3. Select Your Schedule:

- What days and times will you practice?

_____

4. Track Your Progress:

- Note how you feel after each session:
  - ■ Day 1: _____
  - ■ Day 2: _____

5. Reflect on Your Experience:

- How has yoga impacted your physical and mental health?

_____

CHAPTER 8
IMPROVE YOUR SLEEP—UNLOCK BETTER HEALTH AND ENERGY

"Sleep is the best meditation."
— Dalai Lama

The Sleep Struggle—A Personal and Professional Challenge

Of all the health concerns people bring to me, sleep issues are among the most common. And to be honest, this is the area I struggle with the most myself.

I remember one colleague in particular who came to me, frustrated with his sleep. He had trouble falling asleep and staying asleep, and it was starting to affect his energy, focus, and overall well-being.

After chatting about his habits, one thing stood out immediately—he was on his phone until the very minute he tried to sleep.

We started small. First, we tried blue light-blocking glasses to reduce melatonin suppression from screen exposure. That helped a little, but not enough.

Then we took the big step—removing the phone from the bedroom entirely. That was the game-changer.

His sleep still wasn't perfect, but it was significantly better. More energy, improved mood, better focus. He was on the journey toward better sleep, and that alone was a huge win.

This is the reality—small changes can make a big difference, and even though sleep isn't always perfect, working toward better habits will transform your health.

Why Sleep Matters More Than You Think

Sleep isn't just about resting—it's when your body repairs, regenerates, and resets.

✓ Boosts Metabolic Health → Poor sleep increases insulin resistance and cravings for processed foods.

✓ Supports Brain Function → Essential for memory, focus, and decision-making.

✓ Regulates Hormones → Impacts hunger hormones (ghrelin/leptin), testosterone, and growth hormone.

✓ Enhances Immune Function → Sleep strengthens your body's ability to fight infection.

✓ Reduces Risk of Chronic Disease → Poor sleep is linked to heart disease, diabetes, and obesity.

✓ Improves Mood & Emotional Resilience → Lack of sleep increases stress, anxiety, and depression.

Simply put: better sleep = better health, better focus, better energy.

Signs You're Not Getting Enough Quality Sleep

Even if you're sleeping enough hours, your sleep quality might be poor. Here are some warning signs:

✕ Waking up feeling exhausted, even after 7–8 hours.

✕ Struggling to fall asleep or waking up in the middle of the night.

✕ Craving sugar and processed foods throughout the day.

✕ Feeling irritable, anxious, or emotionally drained.

✕ Needing caffeine to function in the morning and afternoon.

✕ Difficulty concentrating or making decisions.

If any of these sound familiar, your sleep could be sabotaging your health—without you even realizing it.

How to Improve Your Sleep: Actionable Strategies

Getting better sleep doesn't have to be complicated, but it does require intentional changes.

1. Control Light Exposure

✓ Morning sunlight → Go outside within 30 minutes of waking up to set your circadian rhythm.

✓ Dim the lights at night → Reduce blue light exposure from screens 1–2 hours before bed.

✓ Use blue light-blocking glasses → Helps prevent melatonin suppression if you must use screens.

✓ Make your bedroom dark → Use blackout curtains or an eye mask for deeper sleep.

2. Keep Your Bedroom a Phone-Free Zone

✓ Charge your phone outside the room → Avoid mindless scrolling before bed.

✓ Use an actual alarm clock → Eliminates the need for a phone on the nightstand.

✓ Create a wind-down routine → Replace screen time with reading, stretching, or journaling.

→ My colleague saw major sleep improvements simply by removing his phone from the bedroom!

3. Optimize Your Sleep Environment

✓ Keep the bedroom cool → Ideal temperature: 60–67°F (16–19°C).

✓ Invest in a comfortable mattress & pillow → Good sleep starts with good support.

✓ Use a white noise machine → Helps block out distractions.

4. Manage Stress Before Bed

✓ Try deep breathing or meditation → Lowers cortisol levels.

✓ Stretch or do light yoga → Releases tension and signals relaxation.

✓ Journal your thoughts → Clears your mind before sleep.

5. Be Consistent with Your Sleep Schedule

✓ Go to bed and wake up at the same time every day (even weekends!).

✓ Avoid long naps → Stick to 20–30 minutes max if needed.

✓ Follow a wind-down routine → Signal to your body that it's time to sleep.

How Sleep Affects Metabolic Health

One of the biggest reasons to prioritize sleep is its impact on metabolism and weight.

When you don't sleep well:

✖ Cravings increase → You're drawn to sugar and processed carbs.

✖ Insulin resistance rises → Blood sugar levels become unstable.

✖ Fat storage increases → Sleep deprivation can promote weight gain.

✖ Energy crashes → Lead to more caffeine and sugar consumption.

When you sleep well:

✓ Hunger hormones are balanced → Fewer cravings.

✓ Insulin sensitivity improves → Blood sugar stays stable.

✓ Your body burns fat more efficiently → Easier weight management.

✓ More energy = better workouts and movement.

Sleep is the ultimate performance enhancer—for your body, brain, and metabolism.

Key Takeaways

✓ Sleep is crucial for metabolic health, energy, and mental well-being.

✓ Poor sleep leads to increased cravings, weight gain, and higher stress levels.

✓ Removing screens from the bedroom can drastically improve sleep quality.

✓ Morning sunlight exposure and a consistent bedtime routine help regulate sleep.

✓ Small changes—like making your room darker and cooler—can have a big impact.

Even if your sleep isn't perfect, working toward better habits will transform your health.

Reflection & Action Plan: Improve Your Sleep

1. What are your biggest sleep challenges? (Falling asleep, staying asleep, waking up tired?)

2. What's one habit you can change this week? (No screens before bed, adjusting room temperature?)

3. How do you feel after nights of great sleep vs. poor sleep?

Jot down your thoughts and set one small goal to improve your sleep.

My Personal Experience

I won't lie—sleep is something I still struggle with. But I've seen firsthand how even small improvements can make a huge difference.

For my colleague, just removing his phone from the bedroom was a game-changer. And for myself, focusing on consistent sleep routines, managing stress, and reducing screen time has helped tremendously.

The takeaway? You don't have to be perfect—you just have to make progress.

Tips for Staying Consistent

✓ Start small → Pick one change at a time.

✓ Track your sleep → Use a journal or sleep tracker.

✓ Be patient → Improving sleep takes time, but the results are worth it.

✓ Prioritize progress over perfection → Every step toward better sleep counts.

Final Thoughts: Sleep is Your Superpower

If you want to optimize your health, energy, and focus, start with better sleep.

It's not always easy, and it won't always be perfect. But every small improvement adds up.

So tonight, try one change—whether it's dimming the lights, leaving your phone outside the bedroom, or going to bed at a set time—and see how it transforms your sleep and your health.

Because at the end of the day, better sleep = better life.

Conclusion

Sleep is not a luxury—it's a necessity.

By prioritizing quality rest, you create a solid foundation for better health, energy, and well-being. Simple changes like a consistent schedule, a calming bedtime routine, and the right supplements can make a world of difference.

Remember, sleep is a self-investment. Whether it's through magnesium glycinate for relaxation, melatonin for travel, or simply a better environment, the benefits of prioritizing sleep will ripple through every aspect of your life.

Start small, stay consistent, and let restful nights guide you toward better days.

Worksheet: Sleep Optimization Plan

Use this worksheet to identify and implement strategies for better sleep:

1. Assess Your Current Sleep Habits:

- How many hours of sleep do you typically get?

_____

- What challenges are you facing (e.g., trouble falling asleep, waking up at night)?

_____

2. Set Your Sleep Goals:

- What time will you go to bed and wake up?

_____

3. Plan Your Evening Routine:

- List three calming activities to incorporate before bed (e.g., reading, stretching, meditation):

_____

4. Optimize Your Environment:

- What changes can you make to your bedroom to improve sleep (e.g., blackout curtains, white noise)?

_____

5. Track Your Progress:

- How do you feel after implementing the changes?

  _____

CHAPTER 9
PRACTICE STRESS MANAGEMENT—FIND YOUR CALM IN THE CHAOS

"You cannot always control what goes on outside,
but you can always control what goes on inside."
— Wayne Dyer

The Power of Perspective: A Mother's Strength in the Face of Crisis

One of the most powerful conversations I've ever had was with a mother of three whose child was sick enough to end up in the ICU.

For any parent, that's an unimaginable situation—the fear, the uncertainty, the emotional exhaustion.

But instead of letting stress consume her, she did something remarkable.

She initiated a gratitude practice to help her navigate the storm.

Even in the midst of one of the most difficult experiences of her life, she made it a point to find something to be grateful for every single day.

She could have spiraled into anxiety, sleep deprivation, and burnout—and many people in similar situations do. But by focusing on gratitude, she maintained her mental clarity, emotional resilience, and physical health.

Today, when you see her, she's still smiling, still full of positivity. She's proof that stress doesn't have to break you—it can make you stronger if you learn how to manage it.

And that's what this chapter is about: not eliminating stress, but learning to handle it in a way that protects your health, sharpens your mind, and helps you thrive—even in the toughest moments.

The Impact of Stress on Your Health

Stress isn't just mental—it has real, measurable effects on your body.

✓ Disrupts Hormonal Balance → Chronically high cortisol levels lead to weight gain, insulin resistance, and increased blood sugar levels.

✓ Weakens the Immune System → Stress reduces your body's ability to fight off infections.

✓ Increases Heart Disease Risk → High stress raises blood pressure and heart rate, increasing the risk of heart attacks and strokes.

✓ Impairs Mental Health → Long-term stress is linked to anxiety, depression, and burnout.

✓ Disrupts Sleep → Stress makes it harder to fall asleep and stay asleep, creating a vicious cycle of fatigue.

✓ Increases Inflammation → Chronic stress fuels systemic inflammation, worsening conditions like diabetes, autoimmune diseases, and chronic pain.

I've seen firsthand how unmanaged stress can land people in the ICU. In extreme cases, stress can cause stress cardiomyopathy—a condition where the heart physically weakens under extreme emotional strain.

If there's one reason to get serious about stress management, this is it—your body depends on it.

Why Stress Management is Non-Negotiable

✓ Protects Your Brain → Reduces brain fog, improves focus and decision-making.

✓ Supports Heart Health → Lowers blood pressure and heart rate.

✓ Boosts Resilience → Helps you handle life's challenges with more ease and confidence.

✓ Promotes Longevity → Chronic stress shortens lifespan, while reducing stress can literally add years to your life.

Stress is inevitable, but suffering from it is optional.

Effective Stress Management Techniques

The key isn't to eliminate stress but to respond to it better. Here's how:

1. Mindfulness & Meditation

✓ Helps quiet racing thoughts and reduces anxiety.

✓ Builds emotional resilience and mental clarity.

- **How to Start:**
  - → Try 5–10 minutes of guided meditation using apps like Headspace or Calm.
  - → Or simply sit quietly and focus on your breath for a few minutes.

2. Deep Breathing (Instant Stress Relief)

Breathing techniques activate the body's relaxation response and lower cortisol levels.

✓ Physiological Sigh

→ Two quick inhales through the nose → Slow, extended exhale through the mouth.

→ Repeat 2–3 times to instantly calm your nervous system.

✓ 4-7-8 Breathing

→ Inhale for 4 seconds → Hold for 7 seconds → Exhale for 8 seconds.

→ Repeat 4–5 times to lower stress and promote relaxation.

3. Exercise & Movement

✓ Exercise lowers cortisol, releases endorphins, and improves mood and resilience.

○ **How to Start:**

→ Go for a brisk 10-minute walk when feeling overwhelmed.

→ Incorporate weightlifting, yoga, or stretching into your routine.

4. Gratitude & Journaling

✓ Shifts your focus away from stress and toward positivity.

✓ Helps you process emotions and gain perspective.

- **How to Start:**

  → Every evening, write down 3 things you're grateful for.

  → Reflect on one challenge you faced and how you overcame it.

5. Social Connection

✓ Talking to someone you trust helps regulate stress and lowers cortisol.

- **How to Start:**

  → Schedule regular check-ins with friends or family.

  → Join a support group or community.

6. Relaxation Techniques

✓ Activities like progressive muscle relaxation, aromatherapy, or listening to music can calm your nervous system.

- **How to Start:**

  → Try progressive muscle relaxation: Tense, then relax each muscle group from your toes to your head.

  → Listen to calming music or nature sounds before bed.

7. **How to Build a Stress-Resilient Routine**

   - **Morning:**

     ✓ Stretch or meditate for 5 minutes.

     ✓ Set an intention for the day.

   - **During Work:**

     ✓ Take deep breathing breaks.

     ✓ Get up and move every hour.

   - **Evening Wind-Down:**

     ✓ No screens 1 hour before bed.

     ✓ Practice gratitude journaling.

     ✓ Read or listen to calming music.

- ◦ **Weekly Self-Care:**

  - ✓ Schedule time for hobbies or outdoor activities.

  - ✓ Take a relaxing bath or spend time in nature.

Consistency is key—small, daily actions add up.

Key Takeaways

- ✓ Stress is inevitable, but suffering from it is optional.

- ✓ Chronic stress damages your body, brain, and metabolism.

- ✓ Simple techniques like deep breathing and gratitude can transform your response to stress.

- ✓ Exercise and social connection are powerful stress relievers.

- ✓ Building daily stress management habits is essential for long-term health.

Reflection & Action Plan: Managing Your Stress

- What are your top stress triggers? (Work, finances, relationships?)

- Which stress management strategies resonate with you? (Meditation, journaling, exercise?)

- How will you integrate stress relief into your routine?

- What's one small change you can make today?

Jot down your answers and commit to one simple action this week.

My Personal Experience

Stress is a constant in my life as an ICU doctor. Long hours, high-pressure decisions, and intense patient situations can take a toll.

But over time, I've learned that stress isn't the enemy— it's how we respond to it that matters.

- ✓ Gratitude journaling has been a game-changer—it shifts my focus from stress to appreciation.

- ✓ The physiological sigh is my go-to during high-stress moments—it calms my nervous system instantly.

- ✓ I've seen how unmanaged stress can literally break the heart (stress cardiomyopathy is real).

If there's one thing I want you to take away from this chapter, it's this:

You have the power to change how stress affects you.

Final Thoughts: Take Control of Your Stress

You can't eliminate stress—but you can build the resilience to handle it better.

Start with one small action today. Whether it's breathing exercises, gratitude, or exercise, find what works for you and make it a habit.

Because when you manage stress effectively, you don't just survive—you thrive.

Conclusion

Stress is an unavoidable part of life, but it doesn't have to control you. By practicing stress management techniques like the physiological sigh, gratitude journaling, and mindfulness, you can transform how you respond to challenges, improve your health, and enhance your overall life quality.

The key is consistency. Whether it's through mindfulness, physical activity, or social connection, find what works for you and make it a regular part of your routine. Small, daily actions can lead to significant improvements in your resilience and well-being.

Remember, stress is not your enemy—it's your body's way of signaling that it's time to take care of yourself. By listening to that signal and responding with intentional strategies, you can thrive even in the face of life's challenges.

Worksheet: Your Stress Management Plan

Use this worksheet to create a personalized plan for managing stress:

1. **Identify Your Stressors:**

   - What situations or activities cause you the most stress?

   _____

2. **Choose Your Techniques:**

   - Which stress management strategies resonate with you (e.g., mindfulness, journaling, breathing exercises)?

   _____

3. **Set Your Routine:**

   - How will you incorporate these techniques into your daily life (e.g., morning meditation, evening journaling)?

   _____

4. **Track Your Progress:**

   - How do you feel after practicing these techniques?

     Day 1: _____

     Day 2: _____

5. Reflect on Your Experience:

- ◦ What's working well, and what adjustments can you make?

_____

CHAPTER 10
BUILD MEANINGFUL CONNECTIONS—THE HEALING POWER OF RELATIONSHIPS

"Connection is why we're here; it is what gives purpose and meaning to our lives." — Brené Brown

---

The Devastating Impact of Isolation

If I learned anything over the course of the pandemic, it was the power and necessity of human connection.

We often talk about nutrition, exercise, sleep, and stress management as pillars of health, but connection is just as important.

I'll never forget some of the patients I cared for during the early days of COVID-19. They had lived full, amazing lives, surrounded by friends and family, but when they became critically ill, they were suddenly isolated from their loved ones.

I saw firsthand how that isolation broke their spirit.

They weren't just physically fighting for their lives—
they were emotionally and mentally depleted from not
seeing the people they loved.

I don't have any data to support this, but it was clear to
me that a lack of connection had a profound impact on
prognosis.

Their will to fight, their motivation to recover—it was fading.

As healthcare providers, we tried our best to step in, to
comfort them, to hold their hands. But we weren't their
spouse, their children, their lifelong friends.

That experience solidified my belief that human
connection is not just a luxury—it's essential for survival
and well-being.

The Science of Connection: Why Relationships Matter for Your Health

We are wired for connection. Research has shown that strong social bonds improve both mental and physical health.

✓ Boosts Immune Function → People with strong social ties have lower levels of inflammation and better immune responses.

✓ Protects Against Chronic Disease → Connection is linked to lower risk of heart disease, stroke, and dementia.

✓ Reduces Stress & Anxiety → Social support helps regulate cortisol levels, reducing the impact of chronic stress.

✓ Increases Longevity → Studies show that people with close relationships live longer.

✓ Improves Mental Health → Strong relationships lower rates of depression, anxiety, and suicide.

✓ Speeds Up Recovery → Patients recovering from illness or surgery heal faster when they have strong social support.

The Consequences of Loneliness

On the flip side, chronic oneliness is as harmful to health as smoking 15 cigarettes a day.

✗ Higher risk of heart disease & stroke

✗ Weakened immune function

✗ Increased risk of dementia

✗ Higher rates of depression & anxiety

✗ Shortened lifespan

The pandemic exposed the silent epidemic of loneliness. It's real, and it's deadly.

How to Strengthen Your Social Connections

Building meaningful relationships doesn't happen by accident; it requires intentional effort. Here's how:

1. Prioritize Quality Over Quantity

✓ It's not about having hundreds of friends—it's about having deep, meaningful connections.

✓ Invest in a few close relationships rather than spreading yourself too thin.

2. Make Time for Loved Ones

✓ Schedule regular meet-ups, calls, or video chats.

✓ Be present—put the phone away and give people your full attention.

3. Engage in Shared Activities

✓ Exercise together → Go for walks, take a yoga class, or play a sport.

✓ Volunteer together → Giving back strengthens relationships and boosts well-being.

✓ Cook or eat together → Meals are a powerful way to connect.

4. Strengthen Your Community

✓ Join a local group → Whether it's a book club, sports league, or religious community, belonging matters.

✓ Reconnect with old friends → A simple text can reignite a valuable friendship.

5. Be the One Who Reaches Out

✓ Many people struggle with loneliness but don't know how to ask for connection.

✓ Take the first step—send the text, make the call, schedule the coffee date.

The Role of Connection in Healing

I've seen firsthand how connection helps people heal.

One patient I'll never forget was an elderly man who spent weeks in the ICU during the pandemic. His condition was serious, but he was still fighting—until he was cut off from his family.

When he could no longer see his wife, talk to his children, or hold his grandchildren's hands, it was as if his spirit left him.

Even though his medical condition hadn't worsened, he stopped engaging, and his prognosis declined.

Contrast that with patients who had strong support systems—those who had families advocating for them, calling them, sending messages of love.

Even when they were critically ill, they had something to fight for.

That's when I realized: medicine can only do so much—human connection is the real lifeline.

Key Takeaways

✓ Connection is just as important as nutrition, exercise, and sleep.

✓ Loneliness is a serious health risk comparable to smoking.

✓ Building strong relationships takes effort, but the rewards are immeasurable.

✓ Simple acts—like checking in on someone—can have a profound impact.

✓ People heal better and live longer when they feel loved and supported.

Reflection & Action Plan: Strengthen Your Connections

• Who are the most important people in your life?

• How often do you connect with them?

• What's one action you can take today to strengthen a relationship? (Call, text, meet up?)

• How do you feel when you spend time with loved ones vs. when you're isolated?

Write down your answers and set a goal to nurture your relationships.

My Personal Experience

I've always known connection was important, but the pandemic changed the way I see it.

As an ICU doctor, I witnessed what happens when people are isolated during critical illness.

- ✓ I saw patients lose their will to fight when they were separated from loved ones.

- ✓ I saw families desperate to be by their loved ones' side but unable to do so.

- ✓ I saw how the presence of loved ones made all the difference in recovery.

This experience reinforced what I already knew:

We are not meant to go through life alone.

Final Thoughts: Connection is Medicine

If you want to live a long, healthy, fulfilling life, you need strong, meaningful relationships.

So don't wait—reach out. Make the call. Send the message. Plan the visit.

Because at the end of the day, health isn't just about the body—it's about the heart.

Conclusion

Health and wellness are not solitary pursuits. By cultivating a supportive community, you can amplify your efforts, stay motivated, and find joy in the process. Surround yourself with people who encourage you, hold you accountable, and share in your journey.

Remember, community isn't just about receiving support—it's also about giving it. By uplifting others, you strengthen your connections and create a ripple effect of positivity and wellness.

Whether it's through joining a group, reconnecting with loved ones, or starting your own community, the relationships you build will become one of your greatest tools for achieving lasting health and happiness. Together, we are stronger.

Worksheet: Building Your Community

Use this worksheet to start cultivating a supportive network:

1. Reflect on Your Current Network:

- Who are the people in your life who already support your health goals?

  _____

- Who could you reach out to for additional encouragement or accountability?

  _____

2. Identify New Opportunities:

- What group activities or events could you join to meet like-minded individuals?

  _____

- Are there online communities you'd like to explore?

  _____

3. Set Community Goals:

- How will you strengthen your existing relationships?

  _____

- What steps will you take to build new connections?

  _____

4. Track Your Progress:

- How has engaging with your community impacted your health and wellness?

  _____

CHAPTER 11
FOSTER HEALTHY HABITS—THE KEY TO LASTING SUCCESS

"We are what we repeatedly do. Excellence, then, is not an act, but a habit."
— Aristotle

A Transformation Through Habit

Sarah was a young nurse and a new mom. With long shifts, sleepless nights, and the demands of caring for her baby, she felt nowhere near her health and wellness goals.

She wanted to get back to her pre-baby weight, but it wasn't just about the scale—it was about feeling strong, confident, and in control of her health again.

At first, the thought of hitting the gym consistently felt impossible. She barely had time for herself. But instead of focusing on perfection, she decided to focus on one simple commitment:

Move every day, no matter what.

- ✓ Some days, this meant brisk walks with her baby in the stroller.

- ✓ Other days, she did exercise snacks—short bursts of bodyweight exercises between tasks.

- ✓ Most days, she made it to the gym for strength training, even if it was just for 30 minutes.

Her husband became her accountability partner, encouraging her to keep going and helping with the baby so she could get her workouts in.

Over time, the results were undeniable.

Sarah not only returned to her pre-baby weight, but she became leaner and stronger than ever before—all because of small, daily habits that became a sustainable lifestyle.

Her success didn't come from a fad diet or an extreme work-out plan—it came from committing, making it easy, and staying consistent.

Why Habits Matter More Than Motivation

Motivation comes and goes. Some days, you feel fired up to eat healthy, exercise, and make great choices. Other days, you don't.

The secret to long-term success? Habits.

When something becomes a habit, it happens automatically—without relying on willpower.

Here's why healthy habits are essential:

✓ Builds Consistency → Keeps you on track, even when motivation is low.

✓ Reduces Decision Fatigue → Eliminates the stress of making choices every day.

✓ Creates Momentum → Small daily actions compound into big results.

✓ Fosters Resilience → A strong foundation makes it easier to bounce back from setbacks.

How to Build Healthy Habits That Stick

1. Start Small

Overhauling your entire lifestyle at once is overwhelming. Instead, start with one small change.

✓ Example: Instead of committing to an hour at the gym, start with 10 minutes of movement per day.

2. Make It Easy

The easier it is to perform a habit, the more likely you are to stick with it.

✓ Example: Lay out your gym clothes the night before or keep healthy snacks within reach.

3. Attach New Habits to Existing Routines

One of the best ways to make a habit stick is to tie it to something you already do.

✓ Example: After brushing your teeth, do a 30-second plank or write one thing you're grateful for.

4. Focus on the Process, Not the Outcome

Instead of obsessing over weight loss or an end goal, focus on the daily actions that will get you there.

✓ Example: Instead of saying, "I want to lose 10 pounds," say, "I will walk for 30 minutes daily."

5. Reward Yourself

Celebrating small wins reinforces habits and keeps motivation high.

✓ Example: After completing a week of workouts, treat yourself to a new book, a massage, or a relaxing bath.

6. Be Patient

Habits take time to form. Setbacks are part of the process—just focus on progress, not perfection.

✓ Example: If you miss a workout, don't quit—just get back on track tomorrow.

Systems Over Goals

Goals are great, but they are short term. A system is what keeps you consistent long after the goal is reached.

✓ Example:

- Goal: Lose 15 pounds.

- System: Strength training 3x per week + meal prepping healthy meals + walking daily.

By focusing on systems, you create sustainable success—even after you reach your goal.

Make Healthy Habits Enjoyable

If you hate your workouts or meal plan, you won't stick to them.

✓ Example: If you dislike running, try dancing, hiking, or boxing.

✓ Make workouts more fun by listening to music or podcasts.

When habits feel enjoyable, not like punishment, they become part of your lifestyle.

The Role of Accountability

✓ Having an accountability partner (like Sarah's husband) makes a huge difference.

✓ Join a community, hire a coach, or find a workout buddy.

✓ Use an app to track workouts or meal prep.

When someone is counting on you, you're more likely to follow through.

Celebrate Small Wins

Every small action counts.

✓ Hit 10,000 steps? Celebrate.

✓ Stuck to your meal plan for a week? Celebrate.

✓ Completed a tough workout? Celebrate.

Celebrating small wins keeps you motivated and reinforces positive behavior.

My Personal Experience

Over the years, I've seen firsthand how habits—not willpower—lead to success.

Example:

- ✓ A patient who struggled with workouts started with just 10 minutes daily.

- ✓ Over time, this grew into a full routine.

- ✓ Their energy, mood, and confidence skyrocketed.

It's not about huge changes overnight—it's about small, sustainable steps that build over time.

Key Takeaways

- ✓ Habits are stronger than motivation—they keep you consistent when motivation fades.

- ✓ Start small, make it easy, and focus on daily actions.

- ✓ Accountability & rewards keep you on track.

- ✓ Systems create long-term success—not just short-term results.

- ✓ Enjoy the journey! When habits are enjoyable, they become a lifestyle.

Final Thoughts: Small Daily Actions = Big Long-Term Success

Sarah's transformation wasn't about perfection—it was about daily commitment.

✓ She didn't wait for motivation—she built habits.

✓ She made it easy, enjoyable, and sustainable.

✓ She became stronger and healthier than ever before.

And that's the key:

◆ Small daily actions lead to big, lasting results.

◆ Stay consistent. Keep moving forward. Your success is in your habits.

Conclusion

Healthy habits are the foundation of lasting health and wellness. By focusing on making small, sustainable changes, creating systems that support your goals, and finding joy in the process, you can build a lifestyle that works for you.

Remember, habits are a journey, not a destination. Celebrate your progress, be patient with yourself, and keep moving forward—one small step at a time. Over time, these small actions will add up to big results, transforming your health and life.

Worksheet: Building Your Healthy Habits

Use this worksheet to create and track your habits:

1. Choose One Habit to Focus On:

- What habit will you build this week?

  _____

2. Break It Down:

- What small steps will you take to start?

  _____

3. Attach It to an Existing Routine:

- When or where will you perform this habit?

  _____

4. Track Your Progress:

  Use the space below to log your efforts:

  Day 1: _____

  Day 2: _____

  Day 3: _____

5. Reward Yourself:

- How will you celebrate your success?

  _____

CHAPTER 12
FINDING YOUR PURPOSE—THE MISSING LINK TO HEALTH AND WELL-BEING

"He who has a why to live can bear almost any how."
— Friedrich Nietzsche

The Connection Between Purpose and Health

In all my years of practicing medicine and studying wellness, one of the biggest realizations I've had is that when you are aligned with your purpose, everything else tends to fall into place. On the flip side, when you are disconnected from your purpose—when your daily actions and values aren't aligned—your health often suffers.

I explored this idea deeply in my previous book, Unapologetic Leadership, in which I talked about the power of leading with purpose. But this doesn't just apply to leadership—it applies to every aspect of life, including your health. When you lack purpose, you're more likely to neglect the very things that sustain you: proper nutrition, sleep, exercise, and mental well-being.

Think about it:

- When you feel unfulfilled in your work or personal life, you might turn to food for comfort, making poor dietary choices.

- If you lack a clear sense of direction, you may experience chronic stress, which disrupts your sleep, metabolism, and energy levels.

- Without purpose, motivation to exercise fades, and unhealthy habits creep in.

Purpose isn't just about having a big mission—it's about aligning your daily activities with what truly matters to you. And when you do that, you naturally start taking better care of yourself.

My Personal Experience: The Pandemic Realization

I came to this realization during one of the most stressful periods of my life—the height of the Omicron wave of the pandemic. At the time, I had recently stepped into the role of Department Head in my hospital, and I was also advocating for schools to stay open to support youth. That decision brought a wave of online criticism—I was attacked, vilified, and heavily scrutinized.

For the first time in my career, I felt afraid to speak up. I hesitated to advocate for what I believed was right, fearing the backlash. And what happened? My health deteriorated.

- I wasn't sleeping.

- I gained weight.

- My eating habits were terrible.

- I stopped exercising.

I was completely out of alignment with my purpose. I felt paralyzed—unsure whether I should continue to use my voice or remain silent. But then, a conversation with Jodi Wilding, one of our guests on the podcast, changed everything.

She spoke about self-leadership and the importance of aligning daily activities with purpose. That hit me hard. I realized that my purpose wasn't about seeking approval—it was about being there for my patients, hearing their stories, relieving suffering, and advocating for what I believed was right.

When I started reconnecting with my purpose, everything started to improve:

- I felt less fear about speaking my mind.

- My stress levels dropped.

- I started exercising again.

- My nutrition and sleep improved.

This was a powerful lesson: When you realign with your purpose, your health naturally follows.

The Story of My Friend—From Unemployment to Purpose

Another powerful example comes from a friend of mine. He lost his job and remained unemployed for an extended period. The impact on his health was profound:

- He gained 30–40 pounds.

- He barely left the house.

- His sleep was so disrupted that he was diagnosed with obstructive sleep apnea.

His life was spiraling, not just because of the job loss, but because he had lost his sense of purpose.

Then, something changed—he found a job that aligned with his core values. Within months, it was like the clouds had lifted:

- He started exercising again.

- He reconnected with his family.

- He met an incredible woman who shared his values and supported his growth.

Today, they have a beautiful family, and he's in a far better place—mentally, emotionally, and physically. All because he found his purpose again.

How to Discover and Align with Your Purpose

Finding your purpose isn't about having all the answers—it's about understanding what truly matters to you and making sure your daily life reflects that.

Here are some steps to help you identify and align with your purpose:

1. Identify Your Core Values

Your purpose is often rooted in your values. Ask yourself:

- What do I truly care about?

- What kind of person do I want to be?

- What activities make me feel the most fulfilled?

2. Reflect on Times You Felt Most Alive

Think back to moments when you felt deeply engaged and fulfilled. What were you doing? Who were you helping?

3. Define Your Personal Mission

- What impact do you want to have on the world?

- How do you want to contribute to the lives of others?

- What legacy do you want to leave behind?

4. Align Your Daily Habits with Your Purpose

Once you have a sense of your purpose, ensure your daily habits reflect it. If health is important to you, structure your day to prioritize exercise, good nutrition, and rest. If family is a core value, dedicate time to meaningful connections.

5. Remove What Doesn't Serve Your Purpose

Eliminate habits, relationships, or commitments that pull you away from what truly matters. This might mean setting boundaries, stepping away from toxic environments, or reducing distractions.

6. Find a Supportive Community

Surround yourself with people who encourage and align with your purpose. Whether they're mentors, like-minded friends, or a professional network, those in your environment play a huge role in your success.

Conclusion: Living with Purpose, Thriving in Health

Your health is deeply intertwined with your sense of purpose. When you're disconnected from what truly matters to you, your habits, energy, and well-being suffer. But when you align your daily actions with your purpose, everything starts to shift in the right direction.

This isn't about being perfect—it's about being intentional. It's about knowing what matters, making small adjustments, and staying committed to living in alignment with your values.

Health is more than what you eat, how you sleep, or how much you exercise—it's about living a meaningful, purpose-driven life. And when you do that, everything else starts to fall into place.

Find your purpose. Live with intention. Thrive in health.

Worksheet: Aligning Your Health with Your Purpose

Use this worksheet to reflect on your purpose and take actionable steps toward aligning your life with it.

Step 1: Identify Your Values

- List 3–5 core values that matter most to you (e.g., health, family, leadership, service):

1. _____

2. _____

3. _____

4. _____

5. _____

Step 2: Define Your Purpose

- What impact do I want to have on the world?

_____

- How do I want to contribute to the lives of others?

_____

- What makes me feel most alive?

_____

Step 3: Assess Your Daily Habits

- Are my daily actions aligned with my values? (Yes/No)

- What 3 things can I change today to realign with my purpose?

1. _____

2. _____

3. _____

Step 4: Create an Action Plan

- What's one habit I can start today to reinforce my purpose?

- Who in my life can support me in this journey?

- What obstacles might get in the way, and how will I overcome them?

CHAPTER 13
SUPPLEMENTS—ENHANCING YOUR HEALTH WHEN FOOD ISN'T ENOUGH

"Let food be thy medicine and medicine be thy food."
— Hippocrates

A Personal Story: The Power of Protein

One of my friends and neighbors was struggling with weight loss and muscle gain. He was moderately overweight, but despite exercising regularly, he wasn't seeing the results he wanted.

After looking at his nutrition habits, it became clear: he wasn't getting enough protein.

We made one simple change—adding a daily protein shake to guarantee he was getting at least 40g of protein first thing in the morning.

We also started tracking his intake, making sure he hit his protein target consistently.

The results?

- ✓ His waist size shrank, but his weight remained the same.

- ✓ He gained lean muscle, improving his strength & metabolism.

- ✓ He felt more energized, stronger, and healthier.

This is a perfect example of how the right supplement, when used correctly, can optimize results without needing drastic changes.

Why Supplements Matter

A balanced diet is the foundation of good health. But in the real world? Life gets busy.

Even with the best intentions, hitting your nutritional targets purely through food can be challenging. This is where supplements can help—not as a replacement for whole foods, but as a tool to fill in the gaps and optimize your health.

I've seen firsthand how targeted supplementation can make a significant difference in muscle recovery, energy levels, immune function, and metabolic health.

I'll also share why we created Gyata Nutrition—a brand designed to provide high-quality, research-backed supplements that support real-life needs.

The Role of Supplements

Supplements are exactly what their name suggests—something that supplements your diet, not replaces it. Whole foods should always be the foundation, but supplements are useful when:

✓ You have higher nutritional needs due to activity levels, age, or specific health conditions.

✓ Some nutrients are hard to obtain through food alone (e.g., vitamin D in winter months).

✓ You need convenience (e.g., protein powder to hit daily intake goals).

Key Supplements for Optimal Health

Here are some of the most beneficial supplements, why they're important, and how they can support your overall health:

1. Magnesium Glycinate

Magnesium is involved in hundreds of bodily functions, but many people are deficient due to modern diets and depleted soil.

✓ Benefits:

- Promotes relaxation and reduces stress

- Improves sleep quality by calming the nervous system

- Supports muscle recovery and reduces cramps

- Helps regulate blood sugar and blood pressure

✓ Why It's Important:

Most people don't get enough magnesium from food. Magnesium glycinate is a highly bioavailable form that is gentle on the stomach and easily absorbed.

2. Creatine

One of the most researched and effective supplements—not just for athletes, but for everyone.

✓ Benefits:

- Increases muscle strength & recovery

- Prevents muscle loss (especially as we age)

- Boosts cognitive function, memory & mental clarity

- Reduces fatigue and improves exercise performance

✓ Why It's Important:

Your body produces creatine, but supplementing can significantly enhance both physical and mental performance.

3. Protein Powder

Protein is crucial for muscle repair, weight management, and overall health—but many people struggle to meet their daily intake.

✓ Bevnefits:

- Helps build & repair muscle
- Supports fat loss by increasing satiety
- Convenient source of high-quality protein
- Great for smoothies, recipes, or post-workout recovery

✓ Why It's Important:

While whole foods like chicken, fish, and legumes are ideal, protein powder offers unmatched convenience—especially post-workout or for busy individuals.

4. Fish Oil (Omega-3s)

Omega-3s are essential fatty acids that reduce inflammation, improve brain health, and support heart function.

✓ Benefits:

- Lowers triglycerides & blood pressure

- Reduces chronic inflammation

- Enhances brain health, memory, and mood

- Alleviates joint pain & stiffness

✓ Why It's Important:

Unless you're eating fatty fish (like salmon) multiple times a week, a fish oil supplement ensures you're getting enough omega-3s.

Why We Started Gyata Nutrition

At Gyata Nutrition, we recognize that proper nutrition is key to staying out of the ICU, but life happens. We wanted to create high-quality supplements that:

✓ Are backed by research

✓ Support real-life needs

✓ Are free from unnecessary fillers or additives

We don't believe in overloading people with unnecessary products—just the essentials to help you perform, recover, and thrive.

How to Incorporate Supplements

Here's an easy, practical way to work supplements into your daily routine:

✓ Morning Routine:

- Vitamin D & Fish Oil – Take these with breakfast to help with absorption.

- Creatine – Easy to stir into your morning coffee, a glass of water, or your smoothie.

- Collagen – Try mixing it into your tea, coffee, or blending it into a smoothie—whatever works best for your morning flow.

✓ Post-Workout:

- Protein Powder – Great to have after exercise to support muscle repair and recovery. Mix with water, milk, or into a smoothie.

✓ Evening Routine:

- Magnesium Glycinate – Take it in the evening to help your body relax and support better sleep.

Key Takeaways

✓ Supplements fill in nutritional gaps, but whole foods come first.

✓ Creatine, magnesium, vitamin D, protein, and omega-3s are some of the most beneficial supplements.

✓ Gyata Nutrition was created to provide effective, research-backed supplements that fit into real life.

✓ Simplicity is key—focus on what works for you and your goals.

Reflection & Action Plan

• What are your primary health goals? (Muscle growth, better sleep, improved energy?)

• Are there nutrients you struggle to get through food alone?

• Which supplements could support your goals?

• How will you incorporate them into your routine?

Final Thoughts: Supplements as Tools, Not Shortcuts

Supplements won't replace a bad diet, but they can be powerful tools when used correctly.

Find what works for you, stay consistent,
and keep focusing on the fundamentals—movement, sleep,
nutrition, and connection.

Because true health is about building habits that last.

Conclusion

Supplements can be a powerful tool in your health arsenal, but they're most effective when paired with a nutritious diet and healthy lifestyle. By choosing the right supplements for your needs and incorporating them thoughtfully, you can support your body in achieving optimal health.

Remember, it's not about doing everything perfectly—it's about finding what works for you and building habits that last. Supplements are just one piece of the puzzle, but they can make a big difference in your health journey when used wisely.

Worksheet: Optimizing Your Supplement Routine

Use this worksheet to identify which supplements might benefit you and how to incorporate them:

1. Assess Your Needs:

- What are your primary health goals (e.g., muscle growth, better sleep, improved recovery)?

  _____

2. Identify Gaps:

- Which nutrients are you struggling to get through food alone?

  _____

3. Choose Your Supplements:

- Which supplements align with your goals and lifestyle?

  _____

4. Track Your Routine:

- Morning: _____

- Post-Workout: _____

- Evening: _____

CHAPTER 14
PERIMENOPAUSE &
MENOPAUSE—BRIDGING THE
GAP IN WOMEN'S HEALTH

---

*"Advocating for women's health isn't just a women's issue—
it's a healthcare issue, a family issue, a workplace issue, and a
justice issue."*
— Dr. Kwadwo Kyeremanteng

A Personal Awakening: From Bystander to Advocate

If you had told me years ago that I'd be speaking out about perimenopause and menopause, I probably wouldn't have believed you. As an ICU physician—a male one at that—I could have easily ignored the issue, assuming it was outside my lane.

But my perspective changed when I watched my own wife go through early menopause.

At first, the symptoms were subtle but relentless—fatigue, mood swings, poor sleep, and a sense of feeling "off." She wasn't herself, and no diet or exercise seemed to help.

She went to doctors, but the response was frustratingly dismissive:

🚫 "It's just stress."

🚫 "It's normal aging."

🚫 "Maybe you should try an antidepressant?"

But she wasn't depressed—her hormones were shifting.

It wasn't until she started hormone replacement therapy (HRT) that everything changed for the better.

✓ Her energy returned.

✓ She slept better.

✓ She became stronger, fitter, and more like herself again.

✓ Her mental clarity improved, and the fog lifted.

✓ Our family life also felt the positive effects—when she felt good, everything else seemed to flow better.

HRT gave her back the quality of life she had lost, and it made me realize something important:

Millions of women are suffering needlessly—not because there isn't a solution, but because they're being denied access, misdiagnosed, or outright dismissed.

That's why I've made it a mission to advocate, educate, and help change the conversation around menopause—both in medicine and society.

Understanding Perimenopause & Menopause

What's the Difference?

✓ Perimenopause: The transitional phase before menopause, lasting 4–10 years. Symptoms can start in the late 30s or early 40s.

✓ Menopause: Officially diagnosed after 12 consecutive months without a period. The average age in North America is 51.

✓ Postmenopause: The stage after menopause, where symptoms may persist but hormone levels stabilize.

The Overlooked Symptoms of Perimenopause

Many women don't even realize they're in perimenopause because symptoms mimic other conditions.

✓ Fatigue & Brain Fog → Often misdiagnosed as burnout or depression.

✓ Sleep Disruptions → Waking up at 3 AM for no reason.

✓ Weight Gain → Especially around the midsection.

✓ Anxiety & Mood Swings → Sudden irritability, sadness, or panic attacks.

✓ Hot Flashes & Night Sweats → Can disrupt sleep and daily life.

✓ Joint Pain & Muscle Loss → Often dismissed as "aging."

✓ Heart Palpitations → Can be confused with anxiety.

🚨 Many women are dismissed by their doctors, told:

◈ "It's just stress."

◈ "It's part of getting older."

◈ "Try antidepressants."

But this isn't just aging—it's hormonal!

Women deserve better answers, better support, and better treatment options.

Why Menopause Matters Beyond Symptoms

Health Risks of Ignoring Menopause

If menopause is not managed properly, it significantly increases the risk of:

- 🚨 Heart Disease → Estrogen protects the cardiovascular system. Postmenopausal women have higher risks of heart attacks and strokes.

- 🚨 Osteoporosis & Fractures → Estrogen helps maintain bone density. Without it, bones weaken, leading to fractures and hip replacements.

- 🚨 Alzheimer's & Cognitive Decline → Estrogen has neuroprotective effects, and low levels increase dementia risk.

Menopause isn't just about hot flashes—it's about long-term health.

What Can Help?

There are several approaches to managing menopause, and what works best depends on the individual.

1. Hormone Replacement Therapy (HRT)

HRT can be life-changing for many women. It replaces estrogen and progesterone, reducing hot flashes, brain fog, and bone loss.

✓ HRT can reduce the risk of:

- Heart disease
- Alzheimer's disease
- Osteoporosis & fractures

⚠ Should everyone take HRT?

No, but every woman should have the choice.

---

2. **Strength Training & Exercise**

One of the best things women can do during menopause is lift weights.

✓ Builds muscle & prevents bone loss

✓ Increases metabolism (which slows during menopause)

✓ Improves mood & mental clarity

---

3. Sleep Optimization

Menopausal sleep disruptions are brutal, but you can improve them with:

✓ Magnesium Glycinate → Helps relaxation & deep sleep

✓ Blue Light Blocking Glasses → Reduce melatonin suppression

✓ Cold Room & Weighted Blanket → Helps with night sweats & anxiety

---

Why We Partnered with Sanomed Life

In our mission to advocate for and support women in midlife, we partnered with Sanomed Life because they share our vision of empowering women through evidence-based solutions.

- ✓ Science-Backed Menopause Care → Sanomed Life provides high-quality solutions tailored to women's hormonal health.

- ✓ Breaking the Stigma → Their work helps normalize menopause conversations in medicine, workplaces, and society.

- ✓ Better Access to Treatment → Many women struggle to access proper care, and Sanomed Life is helping bridge that gap.

This partnership is about more than just supplements— it's about advocacy, education, and action.

Reflections & Key Takeaways

For Women

✓ Advocate for yourself. Many doctors are not up to date on menopause treatment—do your own research.

✓ You deserve to feel strong, healthy, and energetic. If you feel dismissed, find a doctor who listens.

For Men

✓ Be an ally. Learn about menopause and support the women in your life.

✓ Encourage open conversations—it will benefit your relationship, family, and workplace.

For Employers

✓ Menopause is a workplace issue. Women are leaving their jobs because of untreated symptoms. Support policies that help.

Final Thoughts: The Fight for Justice in Women's Health

For too long, menopause has been ignored, dismissed, and stigmatized.

Women deserve better education, better healthcare, and more options.

They deserve to feel strong, energetic, and in control of their health.

And they deserve allies—both male and female—to fight alongside them.

If you're a woman struggling with perimenopause or menopause—advocate for yourself.

If you're a man, be an ally.

If you're a doctor, get educated and be part of the change.

It's time to break the silence. Because when women thrive, we all thrive.

CHAPTER 15
FINAL THOUGHTS - THE PARETO PRINCIPLE IN ACTION

"Success doesn't come from doing everything.
It comes from doing the right things."
— Unknown

As we close this journey through the key habits and strategies for optimizing your health, it's important to revisit a simple but powerful idea: the Pareto Principle, also known as the 80/20 rule. This principle suggests that 80% of your results often come from just 20% of your actions. When applied to health and wellness, it highlights the importance of focusing on the habits that deliver the greatest impact, rather than spreading yourself thin over too many changes.

This chapter is about making your health journey efficient, sustainable, and aligned with your unique goals. By identifying and prioritizing the most impactful actions, you can maximize your efforts while minimizing overwhelm.

What Is the Pareto Principle?

The Pareto Principle was first observed by Italian economist Vilfredo Pareto, who noticed that 80% of Italy's land was owned by 20% of its population. Over time, this concept has been applied to countless areas of life, including business, productivity, and health.

In the context of wellness, it means that a small number of intentional actions—your 20%—can drive the majority of your results. For example:

- Eating protein-rich, whole foods at every meal might account for 80% of your nutrition improvements.

- Lifting weights and walking consistently could deliver 80% of your fitness benefits.

- Prioritizing sleep hygiene and stress management could significantly improve your energy, mood, and resilience.

The key is identifying which habits and actions create the biggest positive ripple effects in your life.

Identifying Your 20%

Every person is unique, so your 20% might look different from someone else's. The first step is to assess your current health and lifestyle to determine which changes will deliver the greatest return on your effort.

Questions to Ask Yourself:

1. Where am I struggling the most?

- Are you struggling with low energy? Poor sleep? Difficulty managing weight?

- Targeting your biggest pain points can often yield the most noticeable results.

2. What habits are already working for me?

- Build on existing strengths. If you're already walking daily, can you increase your step count or add bodyweight exercises?

3. What changes feel realistic and sustainable?

- Focus on habits that fit into your current lifestyle. Small, sustainable changes often deliver the best long-term results.

4. What has worked for others in similar situations?

- Learning from others' successes can help you identify high-impact actions to try.

Examples of the Pareto Principle in Action

Here's how the Pareto Principle applies across key areas of health and wellness:

1. Nutrition

- The 20%:

    - Prioritize eating protein-rich, whole foods at every meal.

    - Eliminate or significantly reduce processed foods and sugary beverages.

- The 80% Impact:

    - Improved metabolism, better appetite control, and reduced risk of chronic diseases like diabetes.

2. Exercise

- The 20%:

    - Focus on strength training 2–3 times per week and walking daily.

    - Incorporate compound lifts and bodyweight exercises, or short HIIT sessions if you're pressed for time.

- The 80% Impact:

    - Increased strength, better insulin sensitivity, and improved cardiovascular health.

3. Sleep

- The 20%:

  - Create a consistent bedtime routine, limit blue light exposure before bed, and optimize your sleep environment (e.g., cool, dark, and quiet).

- The 80% Impact:

  - Better energy levels, improved mood, and reduced inflammation.

4. Stress Management

- The 20%:

  - Practice mindfulness or gratitude journaling for 5–10 minutes daily.

  - Incorporate deep breathing exercises like the physiological sigh to calm your nervous system.

- The 80% Impact:

  - Lower cortisol levels, improved emotional resilience, and reduced risk of stress-related health issues.

Staying Focused on High-Impact Actions

It's easy to get distracted by trends, fads, or the desire to tackle everything at once. The Pareto Principle reminds us to focus on what truly matters and let go of the rest. Here are some tips to maintain focus:

1. **Keep It Simple**

    Don't over complicate your health journey. Start with one or two impactful habits, master them, and then build from there.

2. **Track Your Progress**

    Use a journal or app to track your habits and measure your progress. Seeing the results of your efforts can reinforce your commitment and keep you motivated.

3. **Reassess Regularly**

    Your 20% might evolve over time as your needs and goals change. Periodically review what's working and adjust your focus accordingly.

4. **Avoid Perfectionism**

    Remember, you don't need to do everything perfectly to see results. Consistency with your most important actions matters more than occasional perfection.

My Personal Experience

As an ICU doctor, I've learned firsthand the importance of focusing on what makes the biggest difference. In the high-stakes environment of the ICU, prioritizing the most critical interventions can save lives. This same principle applies to health and wellness: identifying and focusing on the most impactful actions can transform your life.

The 20% for me includes prioritizing sleep, maintaining a strength training routine, and ensuring I get enough protein daily. These habits provide the foundation for my energy, resilience, and overall well-being. I've also seen how simple, high-impact changes like walking more or improving sleep hygiene can dramatically improve my patients' health outcomes.

One patient I worked with started by simply increasing their protein intake and walking 10,000 steps daily. These two changes—just their 20%—led to significant weight loss, better blood sugar control, and improved energy levels in a matter of months. It's a powerful reminder that small, intentional efforts can lead to big results.

Conclusion

The Pareto Principle is a simple but transformative way to approach your health and wellness journey. By focusing on the 20% of actions that deliver 80% of the results, you can create an effective and sustainable plan.

Remember, health is a journey, not a sprint. By identifying your high-impact actions, staying consistent, and giving yourself grace along the way, you'll be well on your way to a healthier, happier life.

Your health doesn't have to be overwhelming. Start small, stay focused, and trust the process. The results will follow.

Worksheet: Finding Your 20%

Use this worksheet to identify and prioritize your high-impact actions:

1. **What are my biggest health challenges?**

   _____

2. **What habits have worked well for me in the past?**

   _____

3. **What small changes feel realistic and sustainable?**

   _____

4. **Which actions will make the biggest difference for my goals?**

   _____

5. **How will I measure progress and stay accountable?**

   _____

CONCLUSION
YOUR JOURNEY BEGINS NOW

As we close the pages of this book, I want to leave you with a simple but powerful message: your health is in your hands. The strategies we've explored—from increasing protein intake to prioritizing sleep, managing stress, and cultivating a supportive community—are tools designed to empower you to take control of your well-being. But the real work begins now, as you implement these principles and make them part of your daily life.

Remember, you don't have to do everything at once. Start small.

Focus on the habits that resonate with you the most, and build from there. The Pareto Principle reminds us that even a few high-impact changes can lead to extraordinary results. Whether it's lifting weights, walking more, or improving your nutrition, every positive step you take moves you closer to the healthiest, happiest version of yourself.

A Final Word of Encouragement

As an ICU doctor, I've seen how critical prevention is. The habits you adopt today can be the difference between thriving and struggling down the road. While it's never too late to make changes, the earlier you start, the more profound the benefits will be.

This book is not just about staying out of the ICU—it's about living a vibrant, fulfilling life. It's about having the energy to chase your dreams, the resilience to face challenges, and the joy of knowing you're taking care of yourself and those you love.

> Health is a journey, not a destination. There will be days when you fall short, and that's okay. Progress is what matters, not perfection. Celebrate your victories, learn from your setbacks, and keep moving forward.

APPENDIX: THE PRESS METHOD™ SCORECARD

---

*A Simple Framework to Take Control of Your Health_*

Over the years of working in the ICU and in preventative health, one thing has become clear: lasting change happens when you simplify the process. That's why we created the **PRESS Method™**—a practical framework to assess where you are today, identify your biggest opportunities, and focus on one or two key actions that drive the most impact.

What is the PRESS Method™?

PRESS is built around five pillars of prevention:

- **P – Purpose**: Are you clear on why you want to be healthy? Do you have a strong "why" that drives your choices?

- **R – Restoration**: Are you sleeping well, managing stress, and allowing your body to recover?

- **E – Eating**: Are you fueling your body with protein-first meals, whole foods, and balanced nutrition?

- **S – Strength**: Are you building and maintaining muscle through resistance training and movement?

- **S – Social Connection**: Do you have meaningful relationships and a supportive community?

When these five areas are aligned, you create the foundation for energy, resilience, and long-term health.

The PRESS Scorecard

The PRESS Scorecard is a simple self-screening tool.

- For each category, give yourself a score from **1 to 5**.

- **5 = Thriving, 1 = Struggling**.

- Any score of **3 or less** is an area of focus.

PRESS Pillar	Score (1–5)	Notes / Observations
Purpose		
Restoration (Sleep/Stress)		
Eating		
Strength		
Social Connection		

☞ Once you've scored yourself, don't try to fix everything at once. Focus on **one or two areas**. This is where Pareto's Principle—the 80/20 rule—comes in. By targeting the 20% of habits that matter most, you'll unlock 80% of the results.

Case Study: A High-Performing Executive

Let's look at a real example.

A female executive in her mid-40s came to us exhausted and frustrated. She was a driven leader and mother of three, but her health was slipping.

Here's how she scored on the PRESS Method:

- **Purpose (4/5):** Strong—her "why" was crystal clear: to show up for her kids and her team.

- **Restoration (3/5):** Good sleep routine, but work stress sometimes took a toll.

- **Eating (2/5):** Struggled with constant snacking, low protein intake, and was 25 pounds overweight.

- **Strength (1/5):** No strength training at all, despite having access to a gym.

- **Social (4/5):** Supportive friends and strong community ties.

Where we focused:

- We worked with her to design a simple but effective **workout plan**, including resistance training fundamentals, to build strength and confidence.

- We addressed her nutrition by **replacing processed snacks with higher-protein options**, including daily **Gyata Nutrition smoothies** to help curb cravings and stabilize energy.

The results:

- 15 pounds lighter within months.

- Stronger than she had ever been in her life.

- More consistent energy, better focus, and greater resilience in both her family life and career.

This is the power of PRESS: focus on what matters most, and real transformation follows.

Why PRESS Coaching Works

The PRESS Method™ isn't just a framework—it's the foundation of our **coaching program**.

Here's what coaching with us looks like:

- **Personalized PRESS Assessment** → identify your areas of opportunity.

- **Targeted Action Plan** → focus on 1–2 levers that create the biggest results.

- **Accountability & Support** → through one-on-one sessions, tools, and community.

Whether you're an executive, a parent, or a team leader, PRESS Coaching helps you build resilience, avoid burnout, and take control of your health—one step at a time.

Ready to Take the Next Step?

If this appendix resonated with you, I'd love to help you put PRESS into action.

☞ Visit **drkwadwo.ca** to learn more about the PRESS Method™, explore our coaching options, and download your free PRESS Scorecard.

Because prevention isn't just about living longer—it's about showing up as your best self today.

ABOUT THE AUTHOR

Dr. Kwadwo Kyeremanteng is an intensive care physician, healthcare leader, and advocate for healthy living. Passionate about preventing illness rather than treating it, Dr. Kyeremanteng promotes a holistic approach to wellness through nutrition, fitness, stress management, and community engagement. He is the founder of Gyata Nutrition and hosts the Prevention Over Prescription podcast, sharing insights and strategies to inspire healthier lifestyles. Dedicated to innovation in healthcare, he co-founded Lionheart Innovation and co-founded the non-profit organizations Bridges Over Barriers and the Black Medical Collective. Dr. Kyeremanteng resides with his family, dedicated to leading by example in all aspects of life.

Instagram: @kwadcast

LinkedIn: https://www.linkedin.com/in/kwadwo-kyeremanteng/

Website: https://drkwadwo.ca/

Email: kwadcast99@gmail.com

thank you

Thank you for reading my book!

Thank you for taking this journey with me. Writing this book and sharing these insights has been deeply rewarding, and I hope it inspires you to take action. Remember, you are not alone in this process. There's a community of like-minded individuals—friends, family, and even people you've never met—who are on this journey with you. Lean on them, share your wins, and help each other grow.

One thing I've learned through my years in medicine and wellness is this: small, consistent actions can lead to profound transformations. Start today, stay consistent, and trust that your effort will pay off.

To your health and happiness,
Dr. Kwadwo Kyeremanteng

www.ingramcontent.com/pod-product-compliance
Lightning Source LLC
Chambersburg PA
CBHW070112030426
42335CB00016B/2127